KT-149-291

OBSTETRICS AND
GYNAECOLOGY

Commissioning Editor: Ellen Green
Project Development Manager: Janice Urquhart
Project Manager: Frances Affleck
Designer: Erik Bigland
Illustrator: Debbie Maizels, Bruce Hogarth

Problem-based OBSTETRICS AND GYNAECOLOGY

Ian A. Greer
MD FRCP(Glas) FRCP(Edin)
FRCP(London) FRCOG MFFP
*Regius Professor of Obstetrics and Gynaecology and
Head of Division of Developmental Medicine,
University of Glasgow, Glasgow, UK*

Iain T. Cameron
BSc MA MD FRCOG MRANZCOG
*Professor of Obstetrics and Gynaecology,
University of Southampton, Southampton, UK*

Brian Magowan
MB ChB DCH MRCOG
*Consultant Obstetrician and Gynaecologist,
The Borders General Hospital, Melrose, UK*

Ralph N. Roberts
BSc MB BCh FRCP MRCOG MD
*Consultant Obstetrician and Gynaecologist,
The Ulster Hospital, Belfast, UK*

James J.Walker
MD FRCP(Glas) FRCP(Edin) FRCOG
*Academic Head of the Unit of
Paediatrics and Obstetrics and Gynaecology,
St James's University Hospital, Leeds, UK*

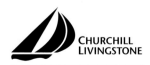

CHURCHILL
LIVINGSTONE

EDINBURGH LONDON NEW YORK PHILADELPHIA ST LOUIS SYDNEY TORONTO 2003

CHURCHILL LIVINGSTONE
An imprint of Elsevier Science Limited

First published 2003

ISBN 0 443 05305 7

British Library Cataloguing in Publication Data
A catalogue record for this book is available from the British Library

Library of Congress Cataloging in Publication Data
A catalog record for this book is available from the Library of Congress

Note
Medical knowledge is constantly changing. As new information becomes
available, changes in treatment, procedures, equipment and the use of drugs
become necessary. The authors and the publishers have taken care to ensure
that the information given in this text is accurate and up to date. However,
readers are strongly advised to confirm that the information, especially with
regard to drug usage, complies with the latest legislation and standards of
practice.

your source for books,
journals and multimedia
in the health sciences
www.elsevierhealth.com

The
publisher's
policy is to use
**paper manufactured
from sustainable forests**

Printed in China by RDC Group Limited

Preface

This book aims to provide a valuable and enjoyable support to clinical teaching in obstetrics and gynaecology. The modern medical curriculum has moved away from the traditional subject-based teaching to a problem-based or problem-orientated approach to learning. Similar changes have occurred in post-graduate medical education. This permits a more realistic approach to the way patients present in the clinical situation and stimulates problem-solving skills. Furthermore such techniques are usually more enjoyable for the teacher and student alike.

In line with this philosophy, this book provides a series of clinical problems with answers, set out by experienced clinicians and teachers. Key topics over the whole of the obstetrics and gynaecology curriculum are covered with a range of difficulty that challenges the student and provides depth as well as breadth of knowledge. Thus we anticipate that the book will also be helpful not only to undergraduates, nurses and midwives, but also postgraduates in their early years of training in obstetrics and gynaecology.

We wish to acknowledge with thanks, the use of the following illustrations from Greer et al 2001 Mosby's Color Atlas and Text of Obstetrics & Gynaecology, Harcourt Publishers, London: Figs 1.1, 3.1, 6.1, 6.2, 6.3, 9.1, 10.1, 10.2, 10.3, 11.2, 12.1 12.2, 19.1, 22.1, 25.1, 25.2, 26.1, 26.2, 29.1, 30.1, 30.2, 32.1, 32.2, 36.1, 38.1, 38.2, 41.2, 44.1, 44.2, 55.2.

I. A. G.
I. T. C.
B. M.
R. N. R.
J. J. W.

Contents

Abbreviations

aPPT	activated partial thromboplastin time
BMI	body mass index
CIN	cervical intraepithelial neoplasia
CTG	cardiotocograph, cardiotocography
CVP	central venous pressure
DIC	disseminated intravascular coagulation
DVT	deep venous thrombosis
FSH	follicle stimulating hormone
GnRH	gonadotrophin releasing hormone
hCG	human chorionic gonadotrophin
HELLP	haemolysis, elevated liver enzymes and low platelets
HSV	herpes simplex virus
INR	international normalized ratio
IUCD	intrauterine contraceptive device
IUGR	intrauterine growth restriction
IVF	in vitro fertilization
LH	luteinizing hormone
LMWH	low molecular weight heparin
MCH	mean corpuscular haemoglobin
MCHC	mean corpuscular haemoglobin concentration
MCV	mean corpuscular volume
PGE_2	prostaglandin E_2
PID	pelvic inflammatory disease
SLE	systemic lupus erythematosus
T_3	tri-iodothyronine
T_4	thyroxine
TSH	thyroid stimulating hormone
UFH	unfractionated heparin
VTE	venous thromboembolism

Fertility and menstrual problems

Primary infertility

A 25 year old woman attends the gynaecology clinic with her partner. They have been trying to conceive for 15 months without success. She has regular menstrual cycles, with bleeding every 28 days.

What initial investigations would you perform?

Based on the knowledge that over 80% of couples would be expected to conceive within 12 months of trying, it would be appropriate to initiate investigations at the request of a couple who have been trying to conceive for 15 months. Specific investigations should be preceded by history and examination. Both the woman and the man should be assessed, irrespective of the likely diagnosis.

HISTORY

A full general medical history should be obtained. Details of previous pregnancies and their outcomes, for the present and previous unions of both partners, should be sought.

In the female history, as in the present case, regular monthly cycles usually indicate regular ovulation. The occurrence of intermenstrual or postcoital bleeding should be noted and investigated as appropriate. A history of abdominal surgery, pelvic infection or ectopic pregnancy might suggest pathology of the fallopian tubes. Previous contraceptive usage, drug history (including tobacco and alcohol), the presence of allergies and relevant genetic, family and social history should also be documented. Enquiry should be made into the woman's immunity to rubella, and an adequate preconception intake of folic acid should be ensured, as folic acid supplementation (0.4 mg daily, or 5 mg daily for women with a previous pregnancy complicated by a neural tube defect) may play a role in the prevention of anencephaly and spina bifida.

In the man, a history of orchitis, epididymitis, torsion, maldescent or varicocele should be sought. Previous sexually transmitted disease, current drug, tobacco and alcohol consumption and the presence of allergies should also be ascertained.

Finally, that the couple enjoy regular intercourse should be determined, and their knowledge of the fertile period of the menstrual cycle should be explored.

EXAMINATION

Besides general medical assessment, physical examination of the woman should include documentation of secondary sexual characteristics and the calculation of body mass index (BMI: kg/m^2, normal range 20–25). Evidence of underlying endocrine disturbance should be sought: goitre, hirsutism and galactorrhoea, for example. Abdominal and pelvic examination should be performed to detect structural abnormality, and a cervical smear should be taken if required.

The purpose of examination of the man is also to exclude underlying general or endocrine disease. The genitalia should be assessed to determine testicular size, volume and consistency, varicocele, epididymal thickening, presence of the vas or scrotal swelling.

INVESTIGATIONS

The aim of initial investigations is to detect ovulation, assess the quality of semen and exclude pelvic pathology in the woman. The woman's rubella status should also be checked.

Assessment of ovulation

Some women experience pain at ovulation, as follicular fluid comes into contact with the peritoneum. Others are aware of changes in the texture of the cervical mucus, which thickens and takes on a clarity and consistency similar to egg white around ovulation.

Further evidence of ovulation can be obtained by daily measurement of basal body temperature. Ovulation is marked by a transient fall in temperature followed by a rise in the luteal phase as a result of the thermogenic action of progesterone. Progesterone itself is secreted by the corpus luteum, which develops from the dominant follicle after ovulation.

More direct evidence of the luteal phase rise in progesterone can be obtained by measurement of the hormone itself. In the face of regular menses (28 ± 7 days), progesterone should be measured in the midluteal phase of the cycle. It is crucial to

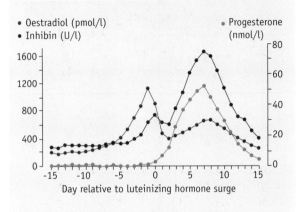

Endocrine profile of the normal menstrual cycle

Fig. 1.1 In the 28 day cycle depicted, progesterone assessment on day 21 would reflect the midluteal phase rise in this hormone. With a longer cycle the length of the luteal phase remains relatively constant; for example, in a 35 day cycle progesterone should be measured on day 28. (Published with permission of Professor S. Hillier and W.B. Saunders)

determine the date of the next menstrual period to be sure that the specimen was obtained at the correct time (Fig. 1.1). Ovulation is suggested when the progesterone concentration is greater than 20 nmol/l. A result between 10 and 20 nmol/l usually indicates incorrect timing of venesection. Other hormonal assessment is not normally necessary in women with regular periods unless there is a suspicion of underlying endocrine disease, or there is a specific complaint such as hirsutism.

Semen analysis

At least two samples should be obtained at an interval of 2–3 months (the normal spermatogenic cycle takes about 70 days). There should be 2–3 days of sexual abstinence before producing the sample, which should be delivered to the laboratory within 1–2 h. According to World Health Organization criteria, normal values include:

Volume	2.0 ml or more
Sperm concentration	20 million/ml or more
Motility	50% or more with forward progression, or 25% with rapid forward progression, within 60 min of ejaculation
Morphology	30% with normal forms

The female pelvis

Diagnostic laparoscopy should be considered to exclude pelvic pathology; at the same time tubal patency is assessed by transcervical instillation of diluted methylene blue dye. Abnormal findings, including endometriosis and pelvic adhesions, should be detailed.

The timing of this invasive procedure has been debated. There is merit in assessing the female pelvis at an early stage in order to make a diagnosis upon which to base a realistic management plan for the couple. In addition, early recourse to laparoscopy should be considered when the history is suggestive of pelvic pathology. If the woman is young (under 30 years), the high spontaneous pregnancy rate within 2 years (about 95%) might suggest that laparoscopy could be deferred when there are no predisposing features.

Should laparoscopy be delayed, hysterosalpingography can be used as a less invasive method of confirming tubal patency; however, this procedure does not provide information about the state of the pelvis, and does not show that the oocyte can gain access to the tube. The other main indications for hysterosalpingography are to demonstrate the anatomy of the cervical canal, to delineate the outline of the endometrial cavity or to determine the level of tubal occlusion as part of the work-up for tubal surgery.

No obvious abnormality is found to account for the couple's delay in becoming pregnant. What further management would you advise?

Although a variety of supplementary investigations are available, including the assessment of sperm–cervical mucus interactions, the measurement of antisperm antibodies or detailed inspection of the uterine tubes by falloposcopy, the results of such investigations do not usually affect the management of the couple in terms of the available treatment options.

With normal ovulation and semen, and patent fallopian tubes, no specific treatment would be indicated for this young couple until they had been trying to conceive for at least 2–3 years, because of the relatively high spontaneous pregnancy rate during this time. Should the couple fail to conceive, the options in the face of 'unexplained' infertility are either to do nothing further, in the hope of spontaneous pregnancy, or to proceed to ovarian stimulation with gonadotrophins (with or without intrauterine insemination of the man's sperm) or assisted conception (in vitro fertilization (IVF) or gamete intrafallopian transfer (GIFT)). The approximate 'take home baby rates' per cycle for these management options range from 2–3% (no treatment, after 3 years unexplained infertility) to 15–20% (IVF). Success rates of 10–20% are quoted after ovarian stimulation and intrauterine insemination. The risks of ovarian hyperstimulation syndrome (OHSS) and multiple pregnancy should always be remembered in women undergoing ovarian stimulation with gonadotrophins (see Case 2).

Secondary infertility

A 33 year old woman attends the infertility clinic having been trying to conceive for 12 months. She has had two pregnancies, which resulted in the birth of her son 3 years previously by emergency caesarean section for fetal distress, and a miscarriage at 10 weeks gestation, following which she required uterine evacuation.

What investigations would you arrange initially?

The three main areas which require investigation are ovulation, semen quality and patency of the fallopian tubes.

Ovulation would be suggested by the presence of regular menstrual cycles (with a menstrual interval of 28 ± 7 days) and the detection of an elevated circulating progesterone concentration (greater than 20 nmol/l — as illustrated in Case 1, a result between 10 and 20 nmol/l usually indicates inappropriate timing of venesection) in the midluteal phase of the cycle. A comprehensive outline of other investigations for the detection of ovulation has already been given in Case 1.

Two semen analyses should be checked at intervals of 2–3 months. If the woman has not changed her partner, the results of the semen analyses should be interpreted in conjunction with the previous evidence of fertilization on two occasions.

Tubal status should be assessed at an early stage in women presenting with secondary infertility, because infection following pregnancy can result in pelvic sepsis and tubal disease. In this case, pelvic pathology could have followed either the caesarean section or the uterine evacuation at the time of the miscarriage. Enquiries should also be made about any previous episodes of pelvic infection (e.g. ruptured appendix or pelvic pain and discharge). Although hysterosalpingography will provide evidence of tubal patency, if adhesions from past infection are suspected, laparoscopy is a better option for viewing the entire pelvis to make the diagnosis. Tubal patency can be determined by insufflation of dilute methylene blue dye at the time of laparoscopy.

Diagnostic laparoscopy confirms the suspicion of previous pelvic infection, with adhesions tethering the ovaries in

the pouch of Douglas and distorting the fallopian tubes. The tubes themselves are grossly dilated. The fimbriae are not visible and there is no passage of methylene blue dye. What treatment options are available? Briefly outline the way in which these treatments are carried out and give the expected success rates.

The treatment options are in vitro fertilization or tubal surgery. IVF would offer the best chance in terms of success rates but its application may be limited by its availability.

IVF

The overall aim of IVF is to fertilize eggs in vitro, creating embryos that can then be placed in the uterine cavity (Fig. 2.1). Initially, the woman is given injections of gonadotrophins (FSH and LH) to stimulate the development of multiple ovarian follicles. In most centres gonadotrophin releasing hormone analogues, such as buserelin, are administered beforehand to 'desensitize' the pituitary gland to prevent premature LH surges, which lead to the need to perform oocyte recovery before the eggs are fully mature. Folliculogenesis is monitored using serial ultrasound scans and serum oestradiol measurements to confirm that stimulation has been successful and to prevent overstimulation and the risk of ovarian hyperstimulation syndrome (OHSS). When the follicles have matured (indicated by a follicle diameter of 16–18 mm and a serum oestradiol concentration of 500–750 pmol/l per follicle) human chorionic gonadotrophin (hCG) is given. This induces ovulation by mimicking the LH surge. The oocytes are then recovered surgically prior to their release from the follicle, which would normally occur 32–36 h after the hCG injection. Oocyte recovery is most often performed under ultrasound monitoring. A needle is passed along a guide attached to a vaginal probe

In vitro fertilization

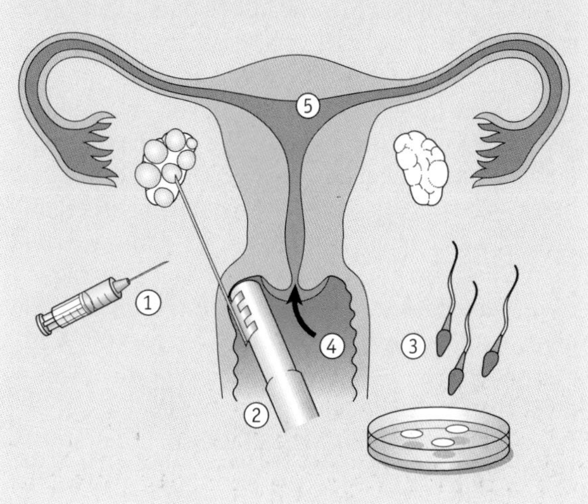

Fig. 2.1 IVF. (1) Ovarian stimulation; (2) transvaginal ultrasound-guided oocyte recovery; (3) in vitro fertilization; (4) embryo transfer; (5) pregnancy.

and pushed through the lateral fornix of the vagina into the ovarian follicle. Aspiration and flushing of the follicle should collect the oocyte and its surrounding granulosa cells. The recovered oocytes are then mixed with a prepared sample of the woman's partner's semen. If fertilization is successful, the fertilized oocyte begins to divide. Embryos are usually transferred to the uterus 48 h after oocyte recovery, by which time they have normally reached the 2–8 cell stage. In the UK, the number of embryos transferred is restricted by law to 3, in order to limit the risk of multiple pregnancy. If implantation occurs, a sensitive pregnancy test measuring hCG should be positive within 2 weeks of embryo transfer.

The 'take home baby rate' for IVF is 15–20% per treatment cycle. The main factors affecting success rates are the woman's age (success rates are considerably reduced when the woman is over 40 years) whether there have been any previous pregnancies and the number of embryos transferred (and their quality).

TUBAL SURGERY

The aim of tubal surgery is to attain patent, mobile tubes that have access to the ovaries. In the present case, surgery might involve adhesiolysis (division of pelvic adhesions) and salpingostomy (creating a new opening for the blocked tube at its fimbrial end). If the tubes are blocked medially, it might be necessary to consider reimplantation of the tube into the myometrium at the cornu. The principles of tubal surgery involve careful handling of tissues and meticulous attention to haemostasis. Consideration should be given to the use of prophylactic antibiotics to prevent infection, and adjuvant treatment with preparations such as intraperitoneal icodextrin solution (Adept®) or ferric hyaluronate gel (Intergel®) to prevent subsequent adhesion formation.

Success rates for tubal surgery vary markedly, but in general they are inversely proportional to the degree of tubal/pelvic damage. It should be noted that although blocked tubes may be made patent by salpingostomy, this does not necessarily mean that the tubes will be able to function normally in terms of either providing nutrient for the early embryo or aiding the transport of gametes or embryos. Furthermore, pregnancy rates after tubal surgery are still dependent upon ovulation and semen quality.

There is an increased risk of ectopic pregnancy after treatment with tubal surgery and, to a lesser extent, IVF. This is probably a reflection of underlying tubal disease, exacerbated by direct tubal manipulation in the case of surgery.

Primary amenorrhoea

A 16 year old attends the gynaecology clinic with her mother. They are both worried that the girl has not yet started to menstruate.

What information would you seek on history and examination?

Enquiry should be made about the development of secondary sexual characteristics; in particular, the girl should be asked about breast development and the growth of axillary and pubic hair. Normal breast growth indicates that the organ has been exposed to oestrogen, whereas axillary and pubic hair development are androgen-mediated events. A general history should also be taken, paying particular attention to family history (such as autoimmune endocrine disease) and noting any episodes of significant weight gain or weight loss.

A general examination should be performed and the girl's height and weight ascertained to calculate her BMI (kg/m^2). Breast development and the growth of axillary and pubic hair should be noted. The pattern of pubic hair and the degree of breast development can be documented semi-objectively using the system developed by Tanner, where a score of 0–5 is allocated, 0 being no development and 5 being the mature female appearance. The characteristic stigmata of Turner's syndrome should be sought (including short stature, sexual infantilism, webbed neck, epican-thal folds and increased carrying angle). The external genitalia should be examined to confirm that they are normal and to exclude clitoromegaly, or blockage to the outflow tract as caused by an intact hymen. Bimanual pelvic examination should be omitted if the girl is not sexually active.

What investigations are warranted at this stage?

The main aim of investigation of amenorrhoea is to exclude abnormality of the hypothalamic–pituitary–ovarian axis and to determine whether the girl has normal female genitalia, both externally and internally. Although pregnancy should always be remembered as an important cause of amenorrhoea, it is more often found in women presenting with secondary amenorrhoea.

The hypothalamic–pituitary–ovarian axis can be screened by measuring the circulating concentrations of FSH, LH, prolactin, TSH, oestradiol and testosterone. Elevated concentrations of gonado-trophins, particularly FSH, would signify ovarian failure, and would be accompanied by a low oestra-diol concentration. Normal or low gonadotrophin concentrations would suggest abnormal pulsatile release of GnRH. The measurement of TSH provides information about thyroid function; both hypothyroidism and hyperthyroidism can result in amenorrhoea.

The girl's karyotype should be determined in order to identify problems such as Turner's syndrome (45,XO), testicular feminization syndrome (46,XY), or pure gonadal dysgenesis (46,XX or 46,XY).

Normal pelvic organs are best demonstrated by ultrasound. It is now rarely necessary to carry out diagnostic laparoscopy to ascertain whether a girl has a normal uterus and ovaries. Although some clinicians would still advocate laparoscopy to view the pelvic organs and obtain an ovarian biopsy in patients with ovarian failure (to distinguish between ovarian failure due to lack of oocytes and ovarian resistance caused by an inability of the ovary to respond to gonadotrophins), others would argue that this is not necessary, as the additional information gained does not alter the patient's management. However, if the ultrasound scan is abnormal, laparoscopy might be indicated to clarify the diagnosis.

The developmental links between the internal genitalia and renal tract should be borne in mind. If ultrasound suggests a uterine abnormality, it would be pertinent to consider renal ultrasound or intravenous ureterography.

Investigations show that the girl has an abnormal karyotype (45,XO/46,XX). Her oestradiol concentration is less than 100 pmol/l. Her FSH and LH concentrations are 45 iu/l and 30 iu/l, respectively. What is the diagnosis?

The girl has Turner syndrome (Fig. 3.1), with a mosaic karyotype. The high gonadotrophin concentrations and low circulating oestradiol concentration indicate inactive ovaries.

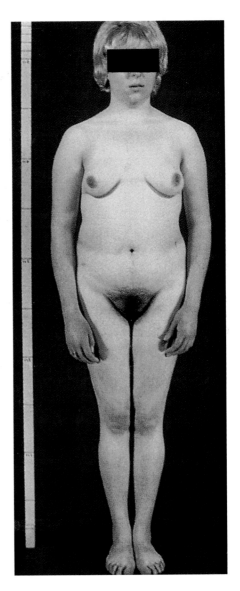

Fig. 3.1 *Features of Turner syndrome. This patient was 162.6 cm (5' 4") in height. One of the commonest forms of mosaicism in Turner syndrome is sex chromatin positive gonadal dysgenesis (XO/XX mosaic). This was the reason for this patient's gonadal dysgenesis. The secondary sexual characteristics were reasonably well developed despite her prime symptoms of amenorrhoea and infertility. (From Tindall VR 1988 A colour atlas of clinical gynaecology. Wolfe Medical Publications Ltd, with permission.)*

How should the patient be managed?

Ensure that the girl and her mother understand what the diagnosis means. Specifically, it should be explained that the girl has an inherited chromosomal abnormality that usually prevents the ovaries from developing normally. The consequences of this are, first that she lacks normal ovarian hormones. The hypo-oestrogenic state causes amenorrhoea (because of lack of the ovarian steroid drive for endometrial development), and is also likely to result in longer term problems, with bone mineral loss and cardiovascular disease. Second, the girl is likely to be infertile because she lacks oocytes. (Note that some individuals with Turner's mosaicism may have normal ovarian function and may be fertile.)

Management should focus on the prescription of hormone replacement for both the development of secondary sexual characteristics and long-term well-being (see below). The girl's prospects for fertility and the follow-up requirements for any inherent medical disorders (such as cardiac and auditory complications) should also be discussed.

Oestrogen replacement is necessary for the development of secondary sexual characteristics and to prevent later problems of osteoporosis and possibly cardiovascular disease. Assuming that the girl has a uterus, oestrogen replacement should be given in combination with progestogen to protect the endometrium from unopposed oestrogen stimulation. For a girl of 16 years of age, combined oestrogen/progestogen is best given eventually as a low-dose combined contraceptive pill, but treatment should begin with a low dose of oestradiol alone to improve initial breast development.

In terms of future fertility, the most reliable option available is oocyte donation as part of an IVF programme. This treatment involves the prescription of oestradiol and progesterone to prepare the endometrium, followed by the transfer into the uterus of embryos created by the fertilization of eggs donated by another woman.

Secondary amenorrhoea

A 25 year old woman attends your clinic complaining that her periods have stopped. She went through the menarche at the age of 15 years and had regular menstrual cycles, with bleeding every 28–33 days until 8 months ago. She is otherwise in good health.

What information would you seek on history and examination?

If the woman is sexually active, the possibility of pregnancy should be borne in mind; thus enquiry should be made about early pregnancy symptoms, such as nausea, breast tenderness and urinary frequency. If necessary the size of the uterus should be assessed by abdominal and bimanual examination, and a pregnancy test should be performed.

A general medical history should be taken, paying particular attention to any recent increase or decrease in weight, and asking whether the woman's previous menstrual bleeding had been spontaneous or the result of withdrawal of exogenous oestrogen and progestogen (such as after treatment with cyclical progestogens for irregular menstruation, or the combined contraceptive pill). The woman should be asked if she has noticed any change in the growth of body hair, which would suggest an increase in the circulating concentration of free androgens, either due to increased androgen production by the ovary or adrenal gland or following a decreased concentration of sex hormone binding globulin (sex hormone binding globulin concentrations are reduced by both hyperandrogenaemia and increased body mass). The woman should also be asked about leakage of fluid or milk from the breasts, which might indicate underlying hyperprolactinaemia caused by a pituitary micro- or macroadenoma, or by a tumour causing pituitary stalk compression.

General examination should be performed and the woman's height and weight documented to calculate her BMI (kg/m^2). The presence of normal secondary sexual characteristics should be noted, as should the presence of hirsutism or galactorrhoea.

Your history elicits the fact that the woman has put on weight and noticed increasing body hair over the last 12 months. Examination shows mild hirsutism, mainly confined to the face, lower abdomen and limbs. Her body mass

index is 37 kg/m². What is the likely diagnosis?

The most common cause of oligomenorrhoea/ secondary amenorrhoea is polycystic ovary syndrome (see Case 9); however, in the present case, excessive weight gain is likely to be the main contributory factor. The mechanism by which changes in body mass cause amenorrhoea is not completely understood, but abnormal pulsatile release of GnRH, in turn due to abnormal input to the hypothalamus from higher brain centres, is thought to play a role. The hirsutism may be explained by the inverse relationship between BMI and sex hormone binding globulin concentrations, resulting in an increased concentration of biologically active free androgen.

What investigations should be performed?

The aim of investigations is to seek a specific abnormality of the hypothalamic–pituitary–ovarian axis, as outlined in Case 3. In contrast to the situation where a woman has not previously menstruated, a complaint of secondary amenorrhoea implies that the woman has had normal female pelvic organs, both internally and externally, and that she has shown evidence of an intact hypothalamic–pituitary–ovarian axis with endometrial growth and regression driven by cyclical ovarian steroid production. Examination or ultrasound scan are not likely to reveal unexpected abnormalities of the internal genitalia, although the scan will permit the assessment of ovarian morphology for the diagnosis of polycystic ovaries (see Case 9). If endocrine assessment reveals no abnormality and the woman fails to menstruate following the prescription of a synthetic progestogen, such as norethisterone or medroxyprogesterone acetate, the possibility of Asherman syndrome should be considered. Asherman syndrome is caused by intrauterine adhesions, most often due to overzealous curettage following early pregnancy loss or term delivery, or tuberculous endometritis. Amenorrhoea is the result of damage to the basal endometrium, preventing endometrial regeneration under the influence of exogenous or endogenous ovarian steroids. Withdrawal of progestogen from an 'oestrogen-primed' endometrium should cause menstrual bleeding. Bleeding will not occur if the woman is 'hypo-oestrogenic' or if the capacity of the endometrium to regenerate is impaired.

The concentrations of FSH, LH, TSH, prolactin, oestradiol and testosterone are within the normal range for a premenopausal woman. What treatment would you recommend?

First, the woman should be encouraged to lose weight, for this action alone might result in the resumption of normal ovarian activity and the return of menstruation.

Next, you should ascertain whether the woman wishes to conceive or whether she merely wants further information and advice about cycle control. If pregnancy is desired, ovulation induction could be considered using the antioestrogen clomiphene citrate; however, it would be preferable for the woman to lose weight before instituting ovulation induction. Not only is treatment more likely to be successful if the woman is slimmer but the pregnancy itself is likely to be less problematic. For example, women who are overweight during pregnancy have an increased risk of pre-eclampsia and gestational diabetes. They may also have bigger babies, with the consequent problems of failed vaginal delivery due to cephalopelvic disproportion or difficult vaginal delivery due to shoulder dystocia.

The woman's partner should be asked to provide a semen sample before the start of ovulation induction to exclude a male factor contribution. If the woman fails to conceive within a few months despite the successful initiation of ovulation, assessment of tubal patency should not be forgotten.

If the woman does not wish to conceive, ovulation induction should not be initiated. Instead, consideration should be given to the prescription of exogenous steroids to induce regular withdrawal bleeding. In this case, as the woman has normal circulating oestradiol concentrations, treatments should be initiated to induce regular withdrawal bleeding in order to protect the endometrium from unopposed oestrogen stimulation and the consequent risks of endometrial hyperplasia, atypical hyperplasia and adenocarcinoma. Cyclical progestogens such as norethisterone (5 mg twice a day) or medroxyprogesterone acetate (10 mg twice a day) could be prescribed for 7–10 days each month. Withdrawal bleeding should occur 2–3 days after discontinuing progestogens if they have been given to women whose endometrium has already been exposed to oestradiol. Alternatively, cycle control can be achieved by the prescription of the combined contraceptive pill, if this is not contraindicated for other reasons. A combined oestrogen–progestogen preparation would be the treatment of choice if the woman were hypo-oestrogenic (suggested by a low circulating concentration of oestradiol or the absence of uterine bleeding after progestogen withdrawal). In this case, the combined oestrogen–progestogen pill would be relatively contraindicated because of the woman's weight.

Menorrhagia in a young girl

A 14 year old girl with irregular, heavy periods presents at your clinic. She went through the menarche at the age of 13 years and this was followed by unpredictable, erratic periods every 2-3 months.

What is the most likely diagnosis?

This girl is likely to have anovulatory dysfunctional uterine bleeding (metropathia haemorrhagica). Anovulatory cycles are common following the menarche prior to final maturation of the positive feedback loop between the ovary and pituitary/hypothalamus. However, pituitary gonadotrophins stimulate ovarian steroidogenesis and the oestradiol so produced promotes endometrial growth. In the absence of ovulation, persistent unopposed oestrogen stimulation eventually results in breakthrough bleeding and unpredictable loss of the functional endometrium.

No further significant features are found after history and examination. What investigations should be performed next?

A full blood count should be carried out to assess haemoglobin concentration and platelet number. A full coagulation screen is not indicated (although a comprehensive family history should be taken), but it should be remembered that bleeding diatheses are a more common cause of menorrhagia in adolescents than in older women. Such abnormalities should always be considered in the adolescent who fails to respond to conventional medical therapy.

As this girl has presented with oligomenorrhoea, it would also be appropriate to screen the hypothalamic–pituitary–ovarian axis by measuring circulating concentrations of FSH, LH, prolactin, TSH, oestradiol and testosterone, as detailed in Cases 3 and 4.

An ultrasound scan of the pelvis should be carried out as an adjunct to clinical examination in young girls for whom bimanual pelvic assessment is inappropriate. The aim of ultrasound should be to exclude lesions of the pelvic organs such as ovarian cysts, or rarely leiomyomata. Curettage is seldom needed to detect organic pathology in adolescents with dysfunctional uterine bleeding. Furthermore, such surgical intervention should be avoided in girls with coagulation defects as curettage can provoke acute bleeding, which may be difficult to control.

What treatment would you advise?

Exogenous steroids should be prescribed to induce regular menstrual bleeding, either in the form of cyclical progestogens or the combined contraceptive pill. Progestogens such as norethisterone or medroxyprogesterone acetate given for 7–10 days in the luteal phase of the cycle (from day 15 or day 19) will promote secretory change in the endometrium, and withdrawal of the steroids will result in predictable, regular menstruation. Alternatively, a low-dose combined oestrogen–progestogen contraceptive pill can be taken.

Besides providing good cycle control, the contraceptive pill will aid in the relief of dysmenorrhoea and is more likely to decrease the degree of menstrual bleeding than will progestogens alone. Treatment should be given for 6–12 months in the first instance and then withdrawn to see whether maturation of the hypothalamic–pituitary–ovarian axis has led to the establishment of a more acceptable pattern of spontaneous menstrual bleeding. If treatment with cyclical progestogens or the combined contraceptive pill is not successful, further investigations must be performed to exclude coagulopathies or underlying organic disorders.

Menorrhagia during the reproductive years

A 36 year old woman complaining of increasingly heavy periods attends your clinic. She has two children aged 10 and 8 years and underwent laparoscopic sterilization 2 years ago. Her periods have worsened since the sterilization procedure.

Outline the main details that should be obtained on history taking.

A comprehensive menstrual history should be taken. In particular the number of days bleeding and the interval between periods should be noted. The woman should be asked whether she has associated dysmenorrhoea. An attempt should be made to determine how heavy her blood loss is, although subjective assessment of the degree of menstrual bleeding is notoriously difficult; for example, there is no relationship between the number of tampons/towels used and objectively measured blood loss. Similarly, although features such as clotting or the use of 'super quality' sanitary protection may suggest heavy blood loss, 50% of women presenting with a subjective complaint of heavy periods have a monthly blood loss within normal limits (less than 80 ml) on objective assessment.

The woman should be asked whether she has had any medical treatment for her periods; if so, details of treatment outcome should be documented. In addition, she should be asked whether she was using the combined contraceptive pill prior to the sterilization procedure. While sterilization itself has not been shown to cause menorrhagia, the combined contraceptive pill will reliably reduce menstrual blood loss by 50%. Discontinuation of the oral contraceptive at the time of sterilization will therefore result in increased menstrual loss.

Besides taking a general history, details should be obtained about the woman's wishes and preferences. For example, she may merely want reassurance that there is no significant underlying disease. Alternatively, she might have decided that she wishes surgical treatment as a definitive cure for her menstrual difficulties.

What signs should be sought on clinical examination?

A general examination should be performed to seek evidence of anaemia or underlying medical disease. Abdominal examination and a bimanual pelvic examination should be carried out to assess the uterus and ovaries. A cervical smear should be obtained if indicated under the cervical surveillance programme.

Examination reveals no specific abnormality. The woman does not appear to be anaemic. There is no abnormal mass in the abdomen, and pelvic examination shows a normal vulva and vagina, a normal cervix (from which a normal smear was taken six months previously), an anteverted, mobile, normal-sized uterus and no adnexal mass. What investigations should be ordered?

A full blood count should be assessed because clinical examination alone is inadequate to exclude iron deficiency anaemia.

The overall aim of investigation is to exclude underlying organic pathology. In a 36 year old woman with regular, heavy menstruation, further investigation is not required before proceeding with treatment if clinical examination is normal. However, if the woman has a history of oligomenorrhoea (implying chronic unopposed oestrogen stimulation of the endometrium with the consequent risk of endometrial atypia), or medical treatment is unsuccessful, further investigation is warranted. This could include a pelvic ultrasound scan to exclude leiomyomata, or hysteroscopy (Fig. 6.1) and endometrial biopsy (or dilatation and curettage) to inspect the endometrial cavity and take a biopsy for histological diagnosis.

What treatment options are available?

If the woman wishes treatment, the options are medical therapy or surgery. Various medical treat-

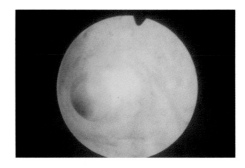

Fig. 6.1 *Hysteroscopic view of the uterine cavity. (Courtesy of Dr M.A. Lumsden)*

ments are available, ranging from drugs that inhibit endometrial prostaglandin synthesis to agents that cause amenorrhoea by suppressing the hypothalamic–pituitary–ovarian axis. The main types of surgical treatment are endometrial resection/ablation or hysterectomy.

A trial of treatment with medical agents (Fig. 6.2) is chosen. What would you recommend?

First-line therapies would be either the prostaglandin synthase inhibitor mefenamic acid (500 mg three or four times a day during menses) or the anti-fibrinolytic agent tranexamic acid (1 g four times a day for the first 3 or 4 days of bleeding). Prostaglandin synthase inhibitors act by diminishing endometrial prostaglandin production. They have been shown to reduce measured menstrual blood loss by about 25% and are relatively free from side-effects in young, healthy women. Tranexamic acid decreases measured menstrual blood loss by about 50% but side-effects, particularly gastrointestinal, are seen more often than with agents such as mefenamic acid.

Another good first-line therapy is the oestrogen–progestogen combined contraceptive pill, as long as the woman has no contraindications to its use (for example, smoking, obesity, previous history/family history of arterial or thrombotic disease). The preparation works by decreasing endometrial prostaglandin concentrations, decreasing endometrial fibrinolysis and promoting endometrial atrophy.

Medical treatments for dysfunctional uterine bleeding

Inhibitors of prostaglandin synthesis	e.g. Mefenamic acid, naproxen
Inhibitors of fibrinolysis	e.g. Tranexamic acid

Hormonal agents	Combined contraceptive pill
	Oral progestogens
	Local progestogens (medicated
	    intrauterine system)
	Danazol
	Gonadotrophin-releasing hormone
	    analogues

Fig. 6.2   Medical treatments for dysfunctional uterine bleeding.

Although cyclical progestogens such as norethisterone or medroxyprogesterone acetate are commonly used for the treatment of ovulatory dysfunctional uterine bleeding, there is little evidence that they are effective at decreasing the degree of menstrual bleeding unless they are given from day 5 of the cycle for 21 days. It is more logical to consider prescription of cyclical progestogens for the treatment of anovulatory dysfunctional uterine bleeding, where drug administration for 7–10 days in the luteal phase of the cycle (from day 15 or 19) will convert unpredictable, irregular bleeding into regular withdrawal bleeding (see Cases 5 and 7).

Recent studies have suggested that local administration of high doses of progestogen by using progestogen-impregnated intrauterine systems may provide a highly effective medical treatment for dysfunctional uterine bleeding. A system impregnated with levonorgestrel (Fig. 6.3) has been shown to reduce measured menstrual blood loss by 80–95%, although troublesome intermenstrual spotting may occur during the first few months of treatment.

Other available agents include the synthetic androgen danazol and gonadotrophin releasing hormone analogues. Although these drugs will reduce the degree of menstrual blood loss reliably (and often cause amenorrhoea), their use is limited because of androgenic and hypo-oestrogenic side-effects, respectively. These agents should not be used as first-line medical treatments for menorrhagia but can be considered in women with intractable menorrhagia who wish to avoid surgery or while they are awaiting surgery.

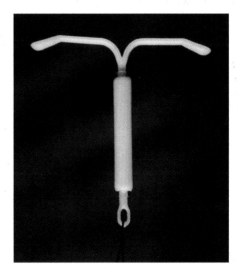

Fig. 6.3   An intrauterine contraceptive system (IUS) impregnated with levonorgestrel.

If the woman had chosen surgical treatment, what advice would you have given her?

The conventional surgical treatment for menorrhagia is hysterectomy. The operation can be performed abdominally or vaginally (the latter with or without laparoscopic assistance). The ovaries can be conserved or removed. In the present case, at the age of 36 years, unless the woman wished to have her ovaries removed, there was a strong family history of ovarian carcinoma or an abnormality was detected at laparotomy, it would be normal to conserve the ovaries to avoid a surgical menopause.

While hysterectomy offers a definitive cure for menorrhagia, it is only appropriate for women who have completed their family and for those who wish to have their uterus removed. For individuals who wish a less invasive surgical treatment, the endometrium can be removed by a variety of techniques (most commonly resection or ablation) by the transcervical route (Fig. 6.4). About 30% of women undergoing these procedures become amenorrhoeic. Of the remainder, most experience a reduction in menstrual bleeding but 10% continue to have menorrhagia. Advantages of this procedure over hysterectomy are that women recover more quickly in terms of their discharge home and return to everyday activities (including work and intercourse). However, follow-up studies

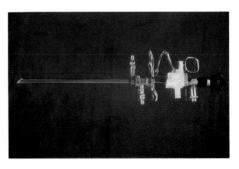

Fig. 6.4 A resectoscope for transcervical endometrial resection. (Courtesy of Dr M.A. Lumsden)

over 2 years have suggested that overall patient satisfaction may be better following hysterectomy. In addition, 20% of women undergoing endometrial ablation/resection will either have the operation repeated at a later date or proceed to hysterectomy. While postoperative morbidity, particularly infection of the vaginal vault or urinary tract, appears to be more common following hysterectomy, endometrial resection/ablation is not without risk. Uterine perforation, which may necessitate emergency hysterectomy, occurs in up to 1% of cases, and care must be taken to ensure that excessive amounts of the fluid used to distend the uterine cavity are not absorbed (with resultant fluid overload and osmotic imbalance).

Menorrhagia during the perimenopause

A 47 year old woman gives a 2 year history of irregular, heavy periods. She went through the menarche at the age of 12 years and always had regular menstrual cycles until 3 years ago. She has had three children, all delivered normally and now in their 'teens. There is no other significant finding on history taking. On examination she is well, but a little overweight. She is not anaemic. Abdominal examination reveals no abnormality and pelvic examination shows a mobile, anteverted, normal-sized uterus.

What is the likely diagnosis?

This woman is likely to have anovulatory dysfunctional uterine bleeding. Anovulation is suggested by the recent history of irregular periods and is a common finding at the extremes of reproductive life, owing to failure of the normal feedback mechanisms between the ovary and the pituitary/hypothalamus.

What further investigations are warranted?

First, a full blood count should be performed. As with any woman presenting with a history of heavy periods, clinical assessment alone is inadequate to exclude iron deficiency anaemia.

In a 47 year old woman with heavy bleeding due to anovulatory cycles, further investigation of the endometrium is required to exclude endometrial atypia as a consequence of unopposed oestrogen stimulation. The least invasive means of obtaining an endometrial sample is by taking a biopsy in the outpatient clinic. An adequate specimen of tissue can usually be obtained without difficulty from parous women, but a disadvantage of the procedure is that it only samples a small percentage of the endometrial surface area. Detection of specific endometrial lesions may be improved by performing endometrial biopsy in conjunction with hysteroscopy. This can also be carried out in an outpatient setting in selected women. Otherwise, a comprehensive assessment of the endometrial cavity can be carried out by hysteroscopy combined with curettage, performed under general anaesthesia in a day-case theatre if the woman is in good general health.

Some authorities would advocate the measurement of circulating concentrations of FSH to determine whether the woman is 'perimenopausal'. While further information can also be obtained by seeking evidence of hot flushes or vaginal dryness on history taking, the woman's management will be the same whether her FSH concentration is normal or elevated.

Your investigations reveal no specific abnormality. What treatment would you suggest?

The most logical treatment would be the prescription of cyclical progestogens, such as norethisterone (5 mg twice a day) or medroxyprogesterone acetate (10 mg twice a day), given for 7–10 days in the second half of the cycle. Withdrawal of the exogenous steroid will result in menstrual bleeding some 2–3 days later, thus converting irregular, anovulatory cycles into regular, predictable menstrual bleeds. The prescription of synthetic progestogens at this dose and interval should also protect the endometrium from hyperplastic change.

In addition, the opportunity should be taken to discuss hormone replacement therapy. Even if the woman does not complain of hot flushes or vaginal dryness, the onset of anovulatory cycles at the age of 47 years is likely to herald the climacteric. The benefits of oestrogen replacement should be explained, in terms of both alleviation of acute symptoms and protection against bone mineral loss.

Fibroids in the uterus

A 42 year old woman is referred to your gynaecology clinic by her general practitioner. She attended her family doctor for a routine cervical smear, at which time pelvic examination suggested that the uterus was enlarged. An ultrasound scan showed that the uterus contained fibroids and was equivalent in size to a 14 week pregnancy.

What are fibroids?

Fibroids, or leiomyomata, are common, benign tumours of the myometrium. They are composed of whorls of smooth muscle and fibrous tissue enclosed in a pseudocapsule. They can be single or multiple, and can vary in size from a few milli-metres to more than 20 cm in diameter. The tumours may be found within the myometrium (intramural), abutting the peritoneal cavity (sub-serosal) or encroaching on the endometrial cavity (submucosal). In addition they can grow on a stalk (pedunculated) extending into the peritoneal cavity or the endometrial cavity (and in some cases may protrude through the cervix). Fibroid growth appears to be dependent upon ovarian steroids; the tumours are common during the reproductive years and regress after the menopause.

Fibroids can undergo a range of pathological changes, including calcification, hyaline change and red degeneration, which normally presents in pregnancy and is thought to be due to impairment of the blood supply to the fibroid as the uterus enlarges. Malignant change is uncommon and is seen in less than 1% of cases.

What are the most common ways in which women with uterine fibroids present?

Larger tumours may present as a pelvic mass or produce symptoms and signs as a result of pres-sure; for example, hydronephrosis due to ureteric obstruction. Fibroids are said to be associated with menorrhagia, dysmenorrhoea, infertility and mis-carriage. However, care should be taken in inter-preting the role of fibroids in these situations by differentiating association from causation. For example, while objective blood loss assessment has confirmed that women with fibroids can present with menorrhagia, fibroid tumours in the myometrium are not necessarily the cause of the endometrial bleeding. Again, there is no clear evi-dence that fibroids cause infertility unless their presence in the cornual region results in tubal occlusion, although it is suggested that submucosal fibroids might impair embryo implantation. The relationship between fibroids and miscarriage is also uncertain, but a clear association has been demonstrated between miscarriage and fibroids greater than 10 cm in diameter. Finally, fibroids are common, and, as in this case, are often found incidentally in otherwise asymptomatic women.

How would you manage the present case?

First, as she is asymptomatic there is no immediate need for treatment unless the woman wants this; however, it would be pertinent to review her (about 6-monthly) and to consider treatment should symptoms develop or should there be a significant increase in the size of the uterus.

If treatment of the fibroids is indicated, the definitive option is surgery. The tumours can be removed by myomectomy, which basically involves shelling them out from the myometrium; however, this can be hazardous in terms of haemorrhage and might necessitate hysterectomy to control the bleeding. In most cases, hysterectomy remains the preferred surgical option for fibroids (Fig. 8.1), with myomectomy being reserved for women who wish to retain their fertility. An exception is the treatment of small to moderate-sized submucosal fibroids, which may be resected by diathermy or laser using a transcervical hysteroscopic approach. Another less radical intervention is uterine artery embolization. While initial outcomes look promising, the results of randomized trials are awaited to judge whether this treatment offers a realistic and effective alternative to more traditional surgical and medical approaches.

Medical therapies can be used to shrink fibroids. The most commonly prescribed preparations are the GnRH analogues (such as buserelin, goserelin or leuprorelin acetate), although recent

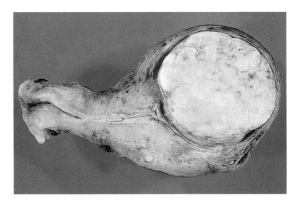

Fig. 8.1 *Uterine fibroid in pathological specimen following hysterectomy. (Courtesy of Dr C. Stewart.)*

studies have suggested that fibroid regression can also follow treatment with antiprogesterones (mifepristone) or high-dose intrauterine progestogens (levonorgestrel impregnated intrauterine system). Maximal reduction in fibroid size is usually achieved within 3 months of treatment with GnRH analogues. The effect is maintained if treatment is continued, but fibroid growth tends to recur after cessation of therapy. Thus, currently available medical treatments do not offer a long-term cure for fibroids. Instead, medical treatment is usually employed as a preoperative adjunct to aid surgery by shrinking the fibroids and reducing uterine blood flow. Medical therapy also offers an alternative for women for whom surgery is contraindicated, although if GnRH analogues are to be given for more than a few months the concomitant administration of exogenous oestrogen–progestogen is advised to alleviate hypo-oestrogenic side-effects.

If the woman remains asymptomatic and there is no evidence of excessive uterine enlargement, spontaneous regression of the fibroids can be anticipated after the menopause.

Oligomenorrhoea

A 22 year old woman presents with a history of heavy, irregular periods. She went through the menarche at the age of 15 years and typically has no more than four or five periods each year.

What further information would you seek by history and examination?

Besides taking a comprehensive general history, specific enquiry should be made about the presence of hirsutism, weight change, treatment with exogenous oestrogens and/or progestogens and family history.

The most likely cause of oligomenorrhoea or secondary amenorrhoea in a 22 year old woman with a long history of irregular periods is polycystic ovary syndrome (see below). As this is usually associated with hyperandrogenaemia, which can result in hirsutism, specific enquiry should be made into the pattern of body hair distribution (see Case 11). Further information about the woman's weight or episodes of significant weight change should be sought, because abnormalities in BMI (normal range 20–25 kg/m^2) are common causes of oligomenorrhoea and amenorrhoea (see Case 4).

As part of the detailed assessment of her previous menstrual pattern, it would be crucial to ascertain whether the woman has ever been prescribed exogenous steroids (for example, in the form of the combined contraceptive pill), which should cause regular menstrual bleeding, masking underlying hypothalamic–pituitary dysfunction.

Finally, further details about family history should be ascertained: both polycystic ovary syndrome and hirsutism have a genetic component.

After the assessment of general features, examination should focus on the determination of BMI, the documentation of body hair distribution, the exclusion of associated endocrine disease (thyroid, adrenal) and the detection of specific pathology in the abdomen and pelvis.

You perform an endocrine profile on day 5 of the menstrual cycle. This reveals a circulating testosterone concentration of 3.2 nmol/l with FSH and LH concentrations of 5 and 17 iu/l, respectively. An ultrasound scan (Fig. 9.1) shows that both ovaries are enlarged, with dense stroma and multiple follicles of 4-8 mm in diameter distributed around the periphery. What is the diagnosis and what is known of the underlying pathophysiology of this condition?

The woman has polycystic ovary syndrome. The precise pathophysiology remains unknown. The

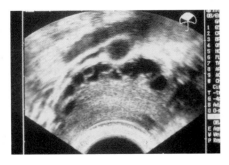

Fig. 9.1 *Ultrasonic scan of a polycystic ovary. Note the dense ovarian stroma and peripherally located follicles.*

disorder is usually associated with anovulation, causing either infertility or anovulatory dysfunctional uterine bleeding, although 25% of normally cycling women have polycystic ovaries on ultrasound assessment. Frequent biochemical features associated with polycystic ovary syndrome are hyperandrogenaemia and an increased circulating concentration of LH. It is not known whether the primary abnormality occurs at the level of the hypothalamus/pituitary or at the level of the gonad. Indeed 'polycystic ovaries' can be seen when the underlying lesion is outside the hypothalamic–pituitary–ovarian axis; up to 5–10% of women with typical polycystic ovaries have excess adrenal androgens because of heterozygosity for 21-hydroxylase deficiency (late-onset congenital adrenal hyperplasia).

Polycystic ovaries can be found in women of all weights but are more often seen in obese than lean women. Overweight women with increased body mass index are more likely to present with hirsutism, which is aggravated by the reduction in sex hormone binding globulin concentrations caused by obesity (leading to an increased circulating concentration of free androgens). Furthermore, many obese women with polycystic ovary syndrome show evidence of insulin resistance. This in turn has important implications for long-term health, increasing the risk of developing type 2 diabetes and cardiovascular disease in later life.

How would you manage this woman's menstrual irregularity?

The options for treatment are the prescription of either cyclical progestogens (norethisterone 5 mg twice a day or medroxyprogesterone acetate 10 mg twice a day) for 7–10 days in the luteal phase of the cycle, or the combined contraceptive pill. Both treatments will provide good menstrual control and protect the endometrium from the unopposed oestrogen stimulation resulting from anovulation. If the woman's BMI is increased, weight reduction should be encouraged. Not only might this alleviate both oligomenorrhoea and hirsutism, but weight reduction will reduce insulin resistance, conferring long-term health benefits.

Advice should also be given about future fertility prospects. With a diagnosis of polycystic ovary syndrome causing oligomenorrhoea and chronic anovulation, the woman is likely to require ovulation induction to help her conceive. The first-line therapy would be antioestrogen treatment with clomiphene citrate or tamoxifen, which should induce ovulation in 90% of cases. It should be emphasized that antioestrogens should only be prescribed for women with anovulation who wish to conceive. For individuals not wishing to be pregnant, cycle control is best achieved using a low-dose combined contraceptive pill, as long as there are no other associated contraindications. Recent studies have advocated insulin-sensitizing agents (such as metformin) as an alternative approach to the treatment of polycystic ovary syndrome. In some women, such treatment appears to reduce hirsutism and improve menstrual patterns.

Menopausal symptoms in a 52 year old woman

A 52 year old woman attends your clinic complaining of hot flushes and night sweats. She has had no period for 14 months.

What other symptoms related to the climacteric might you elicit on history taking?

In addition to vasomotor symptoms, the woman might complain of vaginal dryness (and changes to the vulva, Fig. 10.1), urinary symptoms (including frequency and nocturia) and central symptoms, ranging from anxiety to depression.

What are the other main consequences of lack of oestrogen in the medium and long term?

The main medium to long-term consequences of hypo-oestrogenism are loss of bone mineral and

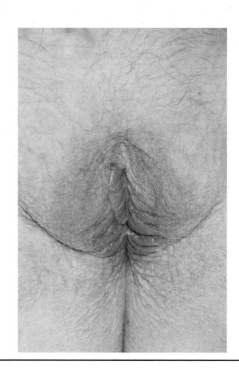

Fig. 10.1   *Postmenopausally the external genitalia undergo change. The skin becomes thin and atrophic, the labia diminish in size and there is a sparsity of pubic hair.*

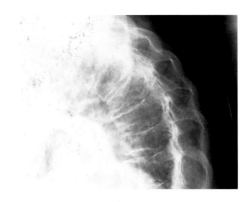

Fig. 10.2 *Osteoporosis leads to fractures in the vertebral bodies and curvature of the spine.*

an increase in the risk of cardiovascular disease. Osteoporosis (Fig. 10.2) is a significant cause of morbidity and mortality in postmenopausal women. There is a loss of calcified trabecular bone resulting in a lowering of the threshold at which fractures can occur. The problems most commonly encountered are vertebral crush fractures, Colles fractures and fractures of the neck of the femur. Slightly built women are most at risk; in obese women the conversion of androgens to estrone in peripheral adipose tissue affords some protection. It should be remembered that peak bone mineralization achieved during the premenopausal years is a crucial determinant of the risk of developing osteoporosis when oestrogen concentrations fall.

Cardiovascular disease is a major cause of morbidity and mortality in developed countries. Premenopausal women are relatively protected from cardiovascular disease when compared with men. The incidence of ischaemic heart disease and stroke increases in women after the menopause, and earlier studies suggested that taking hormone replacement therapy might reduce death rates due to ischaemic heart disease. The precise mechanism by which oestrogen could confer cardiovascular protection is not known. Many studies have suggested that the effect may be related to the action of oestrogens on blood lipids. In addition, oestrogens may have a direct action on vascular endothelium and vascular smooth muscle (or an indirect action via the release of local mediators). That having been said, recent epidemiological studies looking at combined oestrogen–progestogen preparations have cast doubt on the cardioprotective role of hormone replacement therapy.

What treatment would you suggest to control this woman's symptoms?

This woman's symptoms should be improved by the prescription of replacement oestrogen. If she still has a uterus, the oestrogen should be given in combination with progestogen to prevent unopposed oestrogen stimulation to the endometrium, which could result in endometrial hyperplasia, atypia or neoplasia.

Oestrogen/progestogen replacement can be given in a variety of ways. If the steroids are given sequentially, most women experience withdrawal 'menstrual' bleeding. This can vary in degree but in up to 10% of such women blood loss will be excessive (greater than 80 ml per month). Withdrawal bleeding can be limited by administering the drugs in a continuous combined fashion. Hormones are most often given orally (Fig. 10.3), transdermally, or subcutaneously in depot form. Transdermal or subcutaneous administration has the advantage of avoiding first-pass effects in the liver. Although effective at relieving menopausal symptoms, resumption of 'menstrual' bleeding and irregular breakthrough bleeding/spotting are major constraints to compliance with hormone replacement therapy.

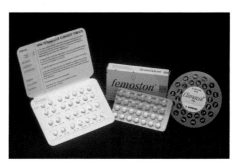

Fig. 10.3 *Hormone replacement therapies come in calendar packs to aid patient compliance. The oestrogenic and progestogenic phases of the pack are distinguished by tablets of different colours.*

While acute symptoms respond quickly to hormone replacement, the effects of exogenous oestrogen on bone mineral metabolism are less rapid. Therapy needs to be taken for 5–10 years (and is best started before the menopause occurs) to show a consistent effect on bone.

What are the potential adverse effects of hormone replacement therapy?

The main adverse effect resulting in discontinuation of therapy is vaginal bleeding, be it regular withdrawal bleeding or unpredictable breakthrough bleeding/spotting. More severe adverse effects are related to the increased predisposition to breast cancer. Although it is difficult to be sure of the precise effect of hormone replacement on breast cancer, because of the difficulties in excluding the many confounding factors, it appears that the incidence of the disease is increased in women who have taken hormone replacement therapy long term when compared with those who have not. However, the relative risk is not large and is more than compensated for by the proven beneficial effects on bone. Nonetheless, women receiving hormone replacement therapy should undergo regular breast assessment (Fig. 10.4), and steroids should be

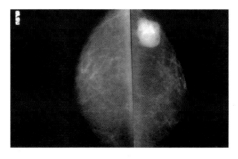

Fig. 10.4 *Mammography showing the presence of a suspicious lesion.*

prescribed with caution for women with a past history of breast cancer or for those with a strong family history of the disease.

A previous history of deep venous thrombosis is not a contraindication to the administration of hormone replacement therapy; however, treatment should be stopped in women who develop an acute thromboembolic event. For individuals suspected to be at high risk of thromboembolism, assessment of thromboembolic status (for example, by measuring antithrombin III and factor V Leiden concentrations and proteins S and C) will help to identify women for whom alternative treatment strategies should be considered or additional surveillance instituted.

Hirsutism in a 32 year old woman

A 32 year old woman is referred to your clinic with a complaint of increased body hair.

What further information should you elicit from the history?

First, you should ask whether the complaint is long-standing or whether it is a recent phenomenon. The rapid onset of hirsutism (Fig. 11.1), particularly if associated with signs of virilism (including loss of body contours, increase in muscle mass and deepening of the voice), would suggest an androgen-secreting tumour or the effects of exogenous steroids. Next, a full menstrual history should be taken. Hirsutism may be associated with oligomenorrhoea, most commonly as a result of polycystic ovary syndrome or weight-related changes. Oligomenorrhoea/amenorrhoea might also indicate underlying endocrine disease (such as hyperprolactinaemia due to a pituitary adenoma, or Cushing syndrome). Enquiries should be made into the woman's general health. She should be asked whether there is a family history of hirsutism and whether she is taking any androgenic medications (such as danazol or androgen-derived progestogens).

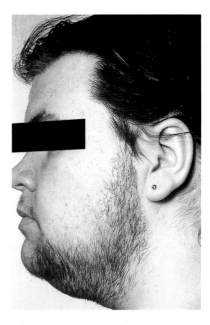

Fig. 11.1 *Hirsutism with excess facial hair. (Courtesy of Professor S. Franks and the Department of Audiovisual Services, Imperial College School of Medicine)*

What specific features would you seek on clinical examination?

The woman's height and weight should be measured to calculate her BMI. A decrease in BMI (as seen in anorexia nervosa) can lead to the widespread appearance of lanugo hair. Increased body mass is often associated with an increased free androgen index, due to reduced circulating concentrations of sex hormone binding globulin, and this in turn predisposes to an increase in male pattern hair growth (see Case 4). General examination should pay particular attention to features of underlying endocrine disease. Abdominal examination should be carried out to exclude the presence of a mass. Clitoromegaly should be sought during pelvic examination.

The pattern of body hair can be documented semiobjectively using the Ferriman–Gallwey scoring system (Fig. 11.2). Briefly, areas of the body, including the upper lip, chin, chest, abdomen and limbs, are allocated a score of 0–4 (with 0 being no hair and 4 being complete cover with dense hair). Nine specific areas are assessed and a score of 10 or more is usually considered abnormal.

What investigations should be carried out?

The overall strategy for investigating hirsutism is, first, to exclude an androgen-secreting tumour, and, second, to determine if there is an excess of androgens. Whether the androgen source is ovarian, adrenal or exogenous (iatrogenic) should also be determined. That having been said, whether the source of excess androgens is ovarian or adrenal, the best medical therapy is the same, namely the prescription of antiandrogens such as cyproterone acetate (see below).

As most women with hirsutism also have oligomenorrhoea, biochemical investigation should be directed towards determining if there are increased circulating androgens and whether there is a specific abnormality of the hypothalamic–pituitary–ovarian axis. Measuring the circulating concentration of testosterone acts as a good screen for hyperandrogenaemia; in the adult woman, the ovary and adrenal contribute equally to peripheral testosterone concentrations. The hypothalamic–pituitary–ovarian axis should be assessed by measuring the circulating concentrations of FSH, LH, prolactin, TSH and oestradiol, as outlined in Case 3.

If the testosterone concentration is elevated (greater than 3 nmol/l), further investigations should be carried out to determine the source of excess androgen. An adrenal site of production would be suggested if there is also an elevation of dehydroepiandrosterone sulphate (DHEAS). If the concentration of 17-hydroxyprogesterone is increased (either basally or after an injection of tetracosactide (Synacthen®)), the diagnosis of late-onset congenital adrenal hyperplasia (heterozygosity for 21-hydroxylase deficiency) can be made. Another way of determining whether increased androgens are secreted by the ovary or the adrenal is to determine the effect of suppressing the hypothalamic–pituitary–ovarian axis with GnRH analogues or the hypothalamic–pituitary–adrenal axis with dexamethasone. A testosterone concentration of greater than 6 nmol/l might suggest an androgen secreting tumour. Computerized tomography (or magnetic resonance imaging) of the ovary, adrenal (and pituitary) may localize the lesion. An alternative technique for identifying the particular site of an androgen secreting tumour is to measure testosterone levels in blood samples obtained by selective venous catheterisation.

What treatment would you recommend for this woman?

Non-endocrine therapies are an important part of the management of excess body hair. Various options are available, ranging from bleaching, shaving, waxing and plucking to electrolysis and laser therapy. Electrolysis often provides the best results, although it is not widely available in many health service settings, and unless the operator has appropriate expertise it can lead to permanent scarring.

The best endocrine treatment for hirsutism is the prescription of antiandrogens, the most commonly used agent being cyproterone acetate, which acts by impairing the way in which testosterone binds to its receptor. Although this drug was

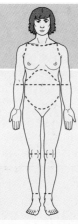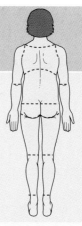

Clinical assessment of body hair growth in women

The Ferriman–Gallwey Score for hirsutism

Site	Grade	Definition
Upper lip	1	A few hairs at the outer margin
	2	A small moustache at the outer margin
	3	A moustache extending halfway from the outer margin
	4	A moustache extending to the midline
Chin	1	A few scattered hairs
	2	Scattered hairs with small concentrations
	3	Complete cover, light
	4	Complete cover, heavy
Chest	1	Circumareolar hairs
	2	Circumareolar hairs with midline in addition
	3	Fusion of these areas, with three-quarter cover
	4	Complete cover
Upper back	1	A few scattered hairs
	2	Rather more, still scattered
	3	Complete cover, light
	4	Complete cover, heavy
Lower back	1	A sacral tuft of hair
	2	A sacral tuft of hair with some lateral extension
	3	Three-quarter cover
	4	Complete cover
Upper abdomen	1	A few midline hairs
	2	Rather more, still midline
	3	Half cover
	4	Full cover
Lower abdomen	1	A few midline hairs
	2	A midline streak of hair
	3	A midline band of hair
	4	An inverted V-shape growth
Arm	1	Sparse growth affecting not more than one quarter of the limb surface
	2	More than 1, but cover still incomplete
	3	Complete cover, light
	4	Complete cover, heavy
Thigh	1, 2, 3, 4	As for arm

Fig. 11.2   *The Ferriman–Gallwey score for hirsutism.*

originally used at a high dose of 50–100 mg daily in combination with oestradiol as part of the 'reverse sequential' regimen, recent studies have suggested that low doses of cyproterone (such as the 3 mg daily found in the combination oestrogen–cyproterone preparation Dianette®) are equally effective; however, it should be noted that improvements in the pattern of body hair are often not seen until treatment has been given for at least 6 months. Cyproterone is contraindicated in women with hepatic disease. Furthermore, liver function tests should be checked before and during treatment (for example, 3–6-monthly with high-dose cyproterone, or annually with Dianette®),

with therapy discontinued if abnormalities of liver function occur. Cyproterone is teratogenic, but this problem is overcome in practice by administering the drug in a contraceptive format. Other antian-drogens with a similar action to cyproterone are spironolactone and flutamide.

Suppression of the hypothalamic–pituitary–ovarian or hypothalamic–pituitary–adrenal axis would seem a logical approach for the treatment of hirsutism due to increased androgen production by the ovary or adrenal, respectively. While such approaches may be beneficial in some patients, treatment with cyproterone, irrespective of the source of androgen, appears to be more effective.

General gynaecology

Vaginal discharge

A 25 year old woman presents with a 3 week history of malodorous vaginal discharge. She describes it as having a fishy smell, which is most noticeable after intercourse.

What is the most likely cause of the discharge?

Vaginal discharge may be of uterine, cervical or vaginal origin. An increase in physiological discharge may be associated with the presence of cervical ectropion, but the most common pathological causes of vaginal discharge are candidiasis, bacterial vaginosis and trichomoniasis. Both bacterial vaginosis and trichomoniasis are associated with a high vaginal pH, and a pH of less than 4.7 virtually excludes these diagnoses. The high pH is due to the production of amines, which cause the fishy smell characteristic of these two conditions. Semen is relatively alkaline, and this explains why the fishy smell is often most noticeable after intercourse. The amine reaction also forms the basis of a simple test in which a drop of discharge is placed on a microscope slide and some potassium hydroxide is added. The easily recognized odour can then be smelled in both of these conditions.

What clinical features would help distinguish between bacterial vaginosis and trichomoniasis (Figs 12.1-12.4)?

Trichomoniasis tends to cause much more irritation that bacterial vaginosis, and thus vulval itch may be a prominent feature. On examination, bacterial vaginosis is associated with a watery grey discharge, while trichomoniasis causes a yellow-green discharge that is often bubbly in appearance. The associated irritation of the cervical epithelium gives it a reddened mottled appearance that has been likened to a strawberry.

Trichomoniasis is caused by a flagellate protozoon, *Trichomonas vaginalis*, which can easily be identified on microscopy of a wet slide preparation. Examination of a wet slide preparation of vaginal fluid in bacterial vaginosis gives the classic appearance of clue cells. These are epithelial cells that have so many adherent bacteria that their borders are obscured.

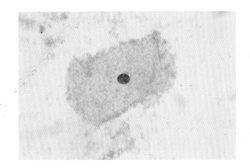

Fig. 12.1 *Cervical smear, Papanicolaou stain: clue cell. This is a squamous cell covered by bacteria, typical of bacterial vaginosis.*

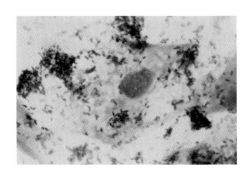

Fig. 12.2 *Gram stain of high vaginal swab showing Gram-negative coccobacilli covering a squamous cell clue cell.*

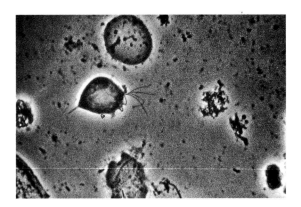

Fig. 12.3 *Microscopy examination of a wet slide preparation of a high vaginal swab showing Trichomonas vaginalis. (Courtesy of Dr Michael McBride.)*

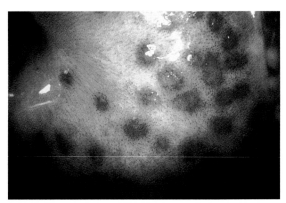

Fig. 12.4 *'Strawberry cervix' typical of trichomoniasis vaginalis. (Courtesy of Dr Michael McBride.)*

What organisms are associated with bacterial vaginosis and what causes it?

A number of organisms may be associated with bacterial vaginosis; the most notable of these is *Gardnerella vaginalis*. Anaerobic organisms may also be involved, such as *Bacteroides* spp., *Mobiluncus* spp. and *Mycoplasma hominis*. Bacterial vaginosis is thus essentially a condition of mixed bacterial overgrowth, and it occurs when the bactericidal effect of the lactobacilli, which form the normal vaginal flora, is lost.

Although not necessarily a sexually transmitted condition, bacterial vaginosis is sexually associated, being found almost exclusively in women who are sexually active. It is commonly seen in association with other sexually transmitted infections, particularly *Trichomonas vaginalis*, *Neisseria gonorrhoea* and *Chlamydia trachomatis*. It is also more common in association with the presence of an intrauterine contraceptive device.

If the diagnosis of bacterial vaginosis is confirmed, what treatment would you suggest?

Bacterial vaginosis is most effectively treated by metronidazole, clindamycin or tinidazole. These may all be given as oral preparations: metronidazole 500 mg b.d. for 7 days, clindamycin 300 mg b.d. for 7 days and tinidazole 500 mg b.d. for 5 days. Metronidazole and clindamycin may also be administered by the vaginal route, metronidazole by twice daily use of 75% gel for 5 days, and clindamycin by nightly insertion of 2% cream for 7 days. There is no evidence that concurrent treatment of the male partner will reduce the rate of recurrence in the female.

Vulval itch

A 60 year old woman presents with a 9 month history of vulval itch.

What additional information would you like to elicit from the history?

It is important to enquire whether there were any precipitating factors or change in routine at the onset of the symptoms. Any exacerbating factors should also be noted. Enquiry should be made into the woman's washing routine, both for herself and her clothes; soap, detergent, deodorants and fragrances commonly cause sensitivity reactions. Enquiry should also be made into all medications, both systemic and topical, that have been used from before the onset of symptoms. Other important questions are whether there are any associated symptoms, such as vaginal discharge, and whether there is any personal or family history of skin disease or atopic conditions.

On examination you note whitened scarring of the vulval skin with resorption of the labia minora. What is the most likely diagnosis?

The most likely diagnosis is lichen sclerosus (Fig. 13.1). This condition has three incidence peaks: in pubertal years, around the time of the menopause and postmenopausal. It has a predilection for genital skin and is associated with

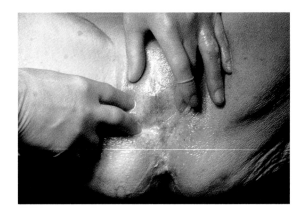

Fig. 13.1 Lichen sclerosis with absorption and adhesion of the labia. (Courtesy of Dr Michael McBride.)

autoimmune disorders. Differential diagnoses are lichen simplex, lichen planus and cicatricial pemphigoid. Features which distinguish lichen sclerosus are resorption of the labia minora and the fact that it never involves mucosal membranes.

How could you confirm the diagnosis?

The diagnosis can be confirmed histologically from a punch biopsy of affected skin. The principal features are loss of the rete pegs, homogeneity of the dermis and, frequently, hyperkeratosis.

What treatment would you prescribe?

The most effective treatment for lichen sclerosus is a potent topical steroid such as clobetasol proprionate (Dermovate®). This should be applied regularly but sparingly, twice daily for 1 month, decreasing thereafter to once daily, with a further decrease or increase in the frequency as dictated by the response. Regular follow up of these patients is recommended as there is an increased risk of developing squamous carcinoma of the vulva.

Vulval ulcer

A 19 year old student attends student health complaining of vulval pain and severe dysuria. She has been in a relationship for a few months but denies having vaginal intercourse. On examination you note inflammation and swelling of the vulva with several ulcers on the labia minora and around the vaginal introitus.

What is the most likely diagnosis?

The most common cause of vulval ulceration in a woman of reproductive years is herpes simplex (Fig. 14.1). Other possible causes of ulceration are a syphilitic primary chancre, chanchroid, Behçet syndrome, severe chemical irritation, or pemphigoid as a result of drug sensitivity.

How might the diagnosis be confirmed?

Characteristic viral cytopathic effects can be detected on cytological examination of scrapings from the base of a fresh ulcer or freshly opened blister. The samples should be smeared on a clear microscope slide and rapidly fixed with a spray fixative or 95% ethanol. The fixed specimen can be stained with Papanicolaou stain, and herpes simplex virus (HSV)-specific fluorescein-conjugated antiserum may be used to identify HSV antigens and to distinguish types I and II.

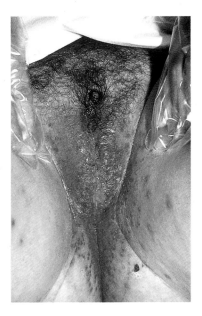

Fig. 14.1 *Primary herpes simplex virus infection. (Courtesy of Dr Michael McBride.)*

HSV types I and II can also be cultured from swabs taken from a clean ulcer or open blister. The swabs can be transported in a transport medium or tissue culture medium and are inoculated onto tissue culture monolayers of human embryonic fibroblasts or monkey kidney cells. Both types of HSV produce characteristic cytopathic changes and the virus can be isolated within 4 days.

Serological studies on acute and convalescent serum can also be helpful in distinguishing primary and recurrent disease.

How may she have contracted this infection?

It is important to appreciate that it is not necessary to have vaginal intercourse to contract genital herpes. The infection may have been transmitted through external genital contact or orogenital contact with a partner who has herpes labialis. In the latter instance it is more likely that HSV type I will be the causative organism.

What is the natural history of this condition?

The initial symptom is usually an itch or tingling sensation which commences 3–9 days after exposure. This progresses quite quickly to the development of erythema and blistering. After 1–2 days the blisters burst, leaving painful ulcers. The ulcers subsequently scab over and heal over the course of 5–10 days.

The herpes simplex virus lies dormant in the dorsal nerve root ganglion, and recurrent attacks may occur when it travels back down the nerve to affect the skin. Recurrence may be precipitated by menstruation, stress or intercurrent illness. In general, recurrent attacks are not as severe as the primary episode, and recurrent attacks of HSV I tend to be less frequent and less severe than those of HSV II.

How would you treat her?

In the early stages of the primary attack it is worthwhile treating systemically with an antiviral agent such as aciclovir or famciclovir. This may reduce the extent of the lesions. Treatment is otherwise along symptomatic lines with adequate analgesia being most important. Dysuria is frequently severe and may lead to urinary retention. Urination can be more comfortable sitting in a bath filled with warm water.

What advice would you give with regard to prevention of future sexual transmission and in relation to childbirth?

The lesions are infective from the moment they appear until they are completely healed. It is also thought to be possible, although relatively unlikely, that transmission of the virus may occur in the absence of current or recent lesions. The safest way to prevent future sexual transmission is thus the use of condoms. In this situation the female condom may be more effective in preventing transmission than the male condom, as it will cover the lesions and reduce the contact of the male scrotum and pubis with the potentially infective areas. When conception is desired, unprotected coitus should not occur within 3 weeks of the development of recurrent lesions.

There is a risk that the virus may be transmitted to the neonate during parturition. This may be associated with a severe systemic primary infection. However, this is unlikely in the absence of active lesions and thus caesarean section is only recommended as a prophylactic measure under these circumstances.

Abnormal cervical smear

You perform a routine cervical smear on a 27 year old parous woman. The cytologist reports severe dyskaryosis.

What would you do next?

The woman should be referred without delay for colposcopy. At the same time as the referral is made, a letter should be sent to the patient to inform her that she will receive an appointment from the colposcopy clinic. It is important that this letter is couched in terms that emphasize the need to attend for colposcopy without causing alarm or unnecessary anxiety.

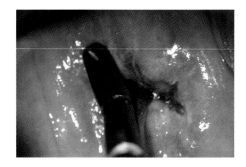

Fig. 15.1 *Directed punch biopsy being taken in an area of acetowhite epithelium.*

What is colposcopic examination?

The aim of colposcopy is to visualize the transformation zone, which is the area of the cervix that undergoes metaplastic change from columnar to squamous epithelium. Colposcopy enables the presence of abnormal cells to be confirmed and their extent to be delineated, and facilitates biopsy from the appropriate region or regions.

A colposcope is essentially a binocular microscope which provides a magnification up to ×40. The cervix should be visualized before the application of any solutions. A green filter can be used to facilitate visualization of the vascular pattern. Acetic acid is then applied to the cervix to assist with identifion of the abnormal epithelium. The abnormal areas become white (acetowhite) and can then be biopsied using punch biopsy forceps (Fig. 15.1).

Histology of the biopsy samples shows CIN III. What do you understand by this term?

CIN is an acronym for cervical intraepithelial neoplasia. CIN III implies that basaloid cells with hyperchromatic nuclei occupy between two-thirds and complete thickness of the epithelium. This is the most severe type of intraepithelial lesion, and, if left untreated, up to 30% will progress to invasive carcinoma.

How can CIN III be treated?

Once the diagnosis of CIN III has been made, the affected areas can be treated by either excision or ablation. Excision has the advantage that tissue is available after the procedure to support the biopsy diagnosis and to confirm that the full extent of the lesion has been treated. Commonly used techniques include large loop exision of the transformation zone (LLETZ), laser conization or a cold knife cone. Hysterectomy is a more radical form of excision but may be appropriate if there are additional indications such as menorrhagia or fibroids.

The ablative techniques are generally less radical and are simpler to perform. However, as no tissue is available for histological examination after the procedure, it is important that a secure histological diagnosis has been made from biopsy samples prior to the procedure. Ablation of the transformation zone may be performed by laser, electrocautery, cryocautery and the misleadingly named cold coagulation, which involves tissue destruction by application of a probe heated to 100°C.

How should this woman be followed up?

Assuming that hysterectomy has not been performed, a follow-up cervical smear should be obtained 6 months after the procedure and, if this is normal, the smear should be repeated at annual intervals thereafter. When five consecutive normal smears have been obtained it would be appropriate to resume routine screening.

If a hysterectomy has been performed a vault smear should be taken at the same intervals as for the cervical cytology.

Pelvic/abdominal mass

A 66 year old women presents with a 3 month history of painless abdominal swelling. On examination you detect a lower abdominal mass, which extends up to the level of the umbilicus. You are unable to get below the mass.

What is the differential diagnosis and what single investigation would be most helpful in assisting with the diagnosis?

The fact that it is not possible to get below the mass on abdominal examination and that it is easily palpable vaginally suggests that it is arising from one of the pelvic organs. The most likely diagnosis is an ovarian cyst. A uterine fibroid could give a similar mass but this is much less likely in the postmenopausal age group, when fibroids have usually regressed.

The most useful investigation for making the diagnosis would be an abdominal ultrasound scan. This would delineate the mass and show its internal structure. It should also be possible to identify the normal pelvic structures.

What features would lead you to believe that the mass is more likely to be malignant than benign?

A short history, with evidence that the mass is growing rapidly, suggests that malignancy is more likely. Hepatomegaly is an adverse feature, as is the presence of ascites; both may be diagnosed clinically or on ultrasound scan. The ultrasound appearance of the cyst itself may also be of help in the preoperative distinction between benign and malignant disease. A benign cyst usually has a thin external wall, and if septae are present they are thin and simple in architecture. A malignant cyst is more likely to have a mixture of cystic and solid areas and septae within the cyst may be thick and fronded. Blood should be taken for the tumour marker CA 125. If this is raised, the cyst is again more likely to be malignant.

How would you manage the case?

The primary purpose of treatment is to remove the cyst intact, or if other organs are involved by malignant spread, to perform maximal surgical debulking. The abdominal incision should be large enough to allow the tumour to be delivered through the wound, so for a large tumour a vertical incision should be used. If ascites is present, a sample should be sent for cytology, and if no ascites is present peritoneal washings should be taken and the fluid sent to cytology. Both ovaries and uterus should be removed and, if there is any suspicion of malignancy, an omentectomy should also be performed to determine whether there has been any omental seeding. The liver should be palpated for evidence of metastases.

The postoperative management will depend on whether the tumour is benign or malignant, and, if malignant, on the type of tumour and its staging. A simplified version of the FIGO (International Federation of Gynaecology and Obstetrics) staging is shown below:

Stage I	Tumour limited to the ovaries
Ia	Tumour limited to one ovary, no ascites
Ib	Tumour affecting both ovaries, no ascites
Ic	Tumour either stage Ia or Ib, but with ascites or positive peritoneal washings
Stage II	Tumour involving one or both ovaries with pelvic extension
IIa	Extension and/or metastases to the uterus and/or fallopian tubes
IIb	Extension to other pelvic tissues including peritoneum
IIIc	Tumour either stage IIa or IIb, but with ascites or positive peritoneal washings
Stage III	Tumour involving one or both ovaries with intraperitoneal metastases outside the pelvis and/or positive retroperitoneal nodes

	Tumour limited to the true pelvis, with proven malignant extension to small bowel or omentum
Stage IV	Tumour involving one or both ovaries with distant metastases, including spread to the liver

Excision of malignant tumours of all stages is generally followed by adjuvant chemotherapy. The most commonly used agents are the platinum derivatives, cisplatin and carboplatin. The progress of treatment and any recurrence of the disease can to some extent be monitored by regular checks on the level of the tumour marker CA 125.

What is the prognosis for survival with ovarian carcinoma and how can recurrent disease be treated?

Long-term survival with ovarian cancer has not increased significantly despite recent advances in treatment. Five year survival rates are 70% for stage I disease, 50% for stage II, 15% for stage III and only 5% for stage IV disease.

Recent improvements in the treatment of recurrent disease have been achieved with the use of paclitaxel, which belongs to a group of drugs called the taxanes. Tumours that have responded poorly to the platinum derivatives occasionally give a prolonged response to paclitaxel.

Postcoital bleeding

A 33 year old woman gives a 9 week history of postcoital bleeding. It is independent of the time of her menstrual cycle and lasts for a number of hours after most occasions of intercourse.

What additional information would you want to acquire from the history?

It is important to ascertain whether there is any unprovoked menstrual bleeding, what form of contraception is being used, and when the last cervical smear was performed.

What are the possible causes of this complaint?

Postcoital bleeding may originate from the uterus, the cervix or the vagina. Uterine causes of this complaint are usually lesions that have prolapsed through the cervix, such as an endometrial polyp or a pedunculated fibroid. The stem of an intrauterine contraceptive device that has become malpositioned may protrude beyond the external cervical os and so cause trauma to the vagina, or indeed the partner's penis, during intercourse.

The most common site of bleeding is the cervix. This may be in association with a simple cervical ectropion or 'erosion'. It may also be due to a cervical polyp (Fig. 17.1), or it may be the

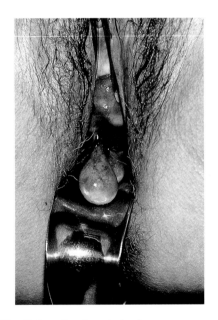

Fig. 17.1   Pedunculated cervical polyp.

presenting symptom of cervical carcinoma. For this reason it is important that the symptom be taken seriously and properly investigated.

More rarely the site of bleeding may be a lesion within the vagina, such as a vaginal tumour. It may also be due to repeated trauma to a previous vaginal laceration or hymenal tear.

On examination you note a cervical polyp 2 cm long and 1 cm in diameter. The tip of the polyp is necrotic and appears to be the site of bleeding. What would you do to exclude other causes of the bleeding, and how would you manage the case?

It is important not to assume automatically that the polyp is the cause of the bleeding and thus omit to exclude other potential causes. If no vaginal lesion is seen, and there is nothing prolapsing through the cervix, the only necessary outpatient investigation would be a cervical smear if this has not been performed since the symptoms began. If an abnormality of cervical cytology was detected this could be treated at the same time as the polyp.

It would be feasible to avulse the polyp using polyp forceps in the outpatient clinic; however, it is wise to destroy the base of the lesion, so it may be better to remove the polyp and either coagulate or excise the base with a wire loop as a day-surgery procedure. If the polyp is emanating from the endocervix, it may be difficult to determine whether it is endometrial or cervical in origin. Under these circumstances, many would perform a hysteroscopy, or at least also explore the uterine cavity with polyp forceps for any endometrial polyps.

When it has been removed, the polyp should be sent for histopathology to exclude malignancy. It is not uncommon for polyps to develop some necrosis, probably due to outgrowing their blood supply, but fortunately malignant change is rare.

Pelvic inflammatory disease

An 18 year old schoolgirl presents to the accident and emergency department with a 24 h history of severe lower abdominal pain accompanied by vaginal discharge, nausea and fever.

What additional information do you wish to elicit from the history?

More information is required about the onset and nature of the pain, its location and whether it has moved, for example from the centre of the abdomen to the right iliac fossa. Enquiry should be made into the presence of associated symptoms, such as nausea, vomiting, urinary symptoms, bowel symptoms and vaginal bleeding. A full menstrual history should be taken and also a sexual history, enquiring about sexual activity, contraception and the possibility of more than one partner. Past medical and surgical history is important, in particular previous appendicectomy or other abdominal surgery.

What signs would you look for on examination?

In addition to fever, the most important findings on general examination are the site of maximum tenderness, and the presence or absence of rebound tenderness and bowel sounds. On speculum examination the most notable findings would be vaginal discharge or bleeding, and on bimanual examination the finding of cervical excitation and tenderness in the vaginal fornices would be highly significant.

How might the diagnosis of pelvic inflammatory disease be substantiated?

Pelvic inflammatory disease is a difficult diagnosis to make on clinical grounds. Not only is this diagnosis liable to be missed, it is also frequently made inappropriately. In these situations it can become a permanent label in a patient's case record and can lead to years of erroneous attribution of symptoms.

Patients with pelvic inflammatory disease will generally have a raised white cell count, but substantive evidence can only be obtained by isolation of responsible organisms or laparoscopy showing salpingitis. Organisms that cause pelvic inflammatory disease are most likely to be isolated from the cervix, but they may also be isolated from the urethra. A Gram stain of a dry slide preparation may show the Gram-negative diplococci responsible for gonorrhoea. Swabs for culture should be placed in Stuart transport medium or plated directly onto chocolate agar.

Chlamydia trachomatis can be isolated from a cervical or urethral swab by direct immunofluoresence, enzyme-linked immunosorbent assay (ELISA) culture on McCoy cells or by molecular techniques such as polymerase chain reaction (PCR) or ligase chain reaction (LCR). As chlamydiae are intracellular parasites it is necessary that epithelial cells are obtained on the swab, so this should be rotated in the cervical os or urethra for a few seconds.

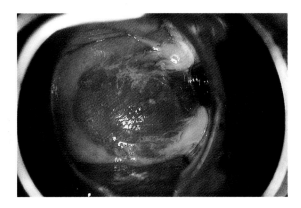

Fig. 18.1   *Gonnoccocal cervicitis. (Courtesy of Dr Michael McBride.)*

How would you treat pelvic inflammatory disease?

A patient with pelvic inflammatory disease who is quite ill should be admitted to hospital and treated initially with intravenous antibiotics. Milder cases can be treated at home with oral antibiotics. The choice of antibiotics is important as they should cover all of the most likely causative organisms and secondary invaders. Chlamydia is the most common causative organism in the United Kingdom; it is sensitive to tetracyclines and erythromycin.

Gonococci (Fig. 18.1) are usually penicillin sensitive. Many secondary bacterial invaders are also sensitive to penicillin, but it is also necessary to cover anaerobic organisms such as *Bacteroides* spp. It is therefore appropriate to give triple antibiotic therapy including a tetracycline or erythromycin, a broad-spectrum penicillin and metronidazole.

A good case can be made for screening the sexual partner for sexually transmitted pathogens. If he is infected, and only the female partner is treated, she is liable to become reinfected. Screening of the male partner is most appropriately performed at a genitourinary medicine clinic suggesting such screening is something that must be handled with sensitivity.

What are the implications of pelvic inflammatory disease for future fertility?

In pelvic inflammatory disease the infection may be confined to the uterus, but it more commonly also involves both fallopian tubes. The risk of long-term damage to the tubes depends both on the causative organism and the time interval before treatment. In general, *Chlamydia trachomatis* causes a more indolent infection than *Neisseria gonorrhoea*. Chlamydial infection is frequently diagnosed late or not diagnosed at all, and is thus associated with a higher risk of tubal damage.

The risk of tubal damage also increases with subsequent infections. The chance of tubal obstruction after a first episode is approximately 10%. This increases to 25% after a second infection and 40% after a third infection. Not only is such tubal damage a cause of infertility but it is also associated with a much greater risk of ectopic pregnancy. The significant increase in chlamydial infections over the last two decades is thought to be one of the causes of the marked rise in incidence of ectopic pregnancy seen during the same time period.

Genital warts

A 22 year old woman presents with a 6 week history of painless lumps on her vulva. There is some associated pruritus but no discharge. On examination you note that she has several condylomata on the labia majora, labia minora and introitus.

What is the causative organism?

Condylomata accuminata, or genital warts (Fig. 19.1), are caused by the human papilloma virus. There are many different types of the virus but those most commonly associated with genital warts are types 16 and 18.

Condylomata lata may be seen on the vulva in cases of secondary syphilis. This, however, is a very rare condition and the condylomata tend to be much bigger and more moist than genital warts.

What is the natural history of the condition?

The incubation period between acquiring the infection and development of warts can be as long

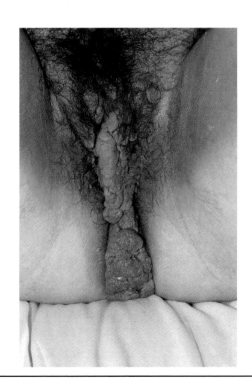

Fig. 19.1 *Genital warts may become extremely extensive in pregnancy. This image shows severe vulval and perianal warts in a pregnant patient, requiring both surgical and medical therapy prior to delivery.*

as 1 year. If left untreated, warts may eventually regress spontaneously, but this can take several years and there may be considerable local proliferation in the meantime. Genital warts tend to proliferate significantly during pregnancy and often regress after delivery.

What methods of treatment are available?

One of the most commonly used treatments is local application of podophyllum (podophyllin). This is a cytotoxic plant extract that is applied to the lesions and left for about 6 hours before being washed off. Several applications at weekly or 2-weekly intervals are usually required. Podophyllin has potential teratogenic effects and its use is therefore contraindicated in pregnancy.

An alternative local application that can be used in pregnancy is trichloroacetic acid. This must be applied very carefully as it causes considerable pain if it gets on normal skin. Once again, several applications may be necessary to effect a cure.

Cryotherapy is often more effective in eradication of an individual lesion but it is very time consuming if multiple condylomata are present. The process involves touching the lesion with a metal probe down which liquid nitrogen is forced to freeze the metal and thus the lesion. Another method for speedy treatment of genital warts is electrocautery. The disadvantage of this treatment is that it requires a general anaesthetic and care must be taken that the heat does not disseminate beyond the lesion and cause scarring.

What advice would you give the woman with regard to the risk of sexual transmission?

There is a risk of infecting the sexual partner until the lesions are totally eradicated. If this process is to take a number of weeks or months, it is unrealistic to expect that the woman will abstain from coitus during this time. She should therefore be advised that, if she does have coitus, condoms should be used on every occasion.

What advice would you give with regard to cervical cytology?

The human papilloma virus has been strongly implicated in the causation of cervical carcinoma. A woman who has suffered from genital warts should therefore have regular assessment of cervical cytology.

Does the condition have any special significance in pregnancy?

The lesions frequently become more numerous during pregnancy, and there is a theoretical risk of infection of the newborn during vaginal delivery. This may be associated with laryngeal papillomas in the infant, but the risk is very small and the presence of genital warts is not generally considered an indication for caesarean section unless the warts are likely to obstruct the second stage of labour or cause problems with repair of the perineum.

Incontinence

A 42 year old woman attends your gynaecology clinic with a history of urinary incontinence.

What are the main types of incontinence encountered in gynaecological practice and what are their pathophysiologies?

The two most common types of incontinence are genuine stress incontinence and detrusor instability, otherwise known as urge incontinence. Genuine stress incontinence occurs when the transmitted pressure within the bladder exceeds the closing pressure of the urethra. Detrusor instability occurs when the bladder muscle contracts without voluntary control, causing loss of urine at inappropriate times.

Other, less common causes of incontinence are retention with overflow, incontinence secondary to a vesical fistula and incontinence secondary to a neurological disorder, such as transection of the spinal cord or multiple sclerosis.

What information would you seek on taking a history?

The history should be directed towards establishing the predominant type of incontinence and whether there are any predisposing factors, and assessing the degree of disturbance to lifestyle. While it must be acknowledged that the history is not always reliable in distinguishing between stress and urge incontinence, it often gives a useful guide. A good starting point is to ask the woman under what circumstances she leaks urine. It is helpful to ask specifically, 'Do you leak urine when you cough, laugh or run?' and 'Do you feel an overwhelming desire to pass urine and leak before you reach the toilet?' Leaking urine on activities that raise intra-abdominal pressure is strongly suggestive of genuine stress incontinence, whereas loss of urine between the desire to void and reaching the toilet is suggestive of urge incontinence. Note that stress and urge incontinence may coexist.

Factors predisposing to stress incontinence are high parity, especially involving large babies and difficult deliveries, obesity and chronic cough, which is often due to smoking.

When establishing disturbance of lifestyle, important points will include whether the woman needs to wear protection throughout the day, how often she changes pads or her underwear, and whether the incontinence restricts her working or social activities.

Other relevant questions are whether the woman is postmenopausal, whether she is taking hormone replacement therapy and whether she has had any previous pelvic surgery.

What specific features would you look for on pelvic examination?

The introitus should be inspected for evidence of vaginal or uterocervical prolapse, as this is a common finding in women with stress incontinence. The woman should then be asked to cough to see if incontinence can be demonstrated. The mobility of the urethra should be assessed, either during coughing or bearing down. It may be necessary to restrain the posterior vaginal wall with either a finger or a Sims speculum to visualize the lower anterior vaginal wall adequately. A bimanual examination should be performed to exclude a pelvic mass, which may be pressing on the bladder. The woman should then be asked to contract her pelvic floor muscles around the examining fingers in order to assess pelvic floor tone.

What initial investigations are appropriate for a woman suspected of having genuine stress incontinence?

In any woman presenting with incontinence it is important to exclude a urinary tract infection. Urinalysis is an adequate screening procedure, but if nitrites or leucocytes are present a midstream sample should be sent for culture.

Another useful investigation is a postmicturition ultrasound scan to exclude chronic retention of urine with overflow incontinence. Urodynamic studies are not always indicated at this stage, but may be helpful if there is doubt about the presence of combined stress and urge incontinence.

What would be your initial management of suspected genuine stress incontinence?

In the majority of cases, the first line of management is pelvic floor exercises. This is usually most sucessful when taught by a trained physiotherapist, who can establish that these exercises are being correctly performed. A woman who has difficulty performing pelvic floor contractions may benefit from the use of a biofeedback probe or electrical stimulation. However, physiotherapy alone will not help the patient with significant prolapse, due to the disturbance of the pelvic floor anatomy. Rather, these women require surgical intervention as a primary procedure. A postmenopausal woman with atrophic changes may benefit from topical oestrogen therapy.

Your patient returns after 4 months of conservative treatment. She reports some improvement in her symptoms, but leaking of urine is still restricting her daily activity. Are there any further investigations which would be of value?

Urodynamic studies may now be helpful to establish that genuine stress incontinence is the correct diagnosis, and that there is no voiding dysfunction. These are two important facts to establish before considering surgical intervention. If there is a significant element of detrusor instability, this may be made worse by surgery. If the woman does not void in the normal way by detrusor contraction in conjunction with urethral sphincter relaxation, operative intervention may result in urinary retention. If the rate of urinary flow is slow, there is also a risk of postoperative urinary retention.

What operations may benefit the woman with isolated genuine stress incontinence?

If there is significant vaginal or uterocervical prolapse, this should be rectified before or at the same time as, a definitive procedure for stress incontinence.

The operation currently considered to be the 'gold standard' is the Burch colposuspension. This operation aims to elevate the bladder neck by suspending it between two sutures that approximate the vagina either side of the bladder neck to the ipsilateral iliopectineal ligament. This procedure has an 80% success rate after 5 years.

Other supension operations are the Marshall–Marchetti–Kranz procedure and the Stamey procedure.

A more recently developed operation is the tension-free vaginal tape procedure. This involves the transvaginal placement of a tape that supports the middle third of the urethra in a sling, the ends of which pass anteriorly between the bladder and the symphysis pubis to emerge at the skin on the mons pubis 2–4 cm lateral to the midline. The high coefficient of friction of the tape means that it does not need to be sutured in place. In the resting state it does not apply any pressure on the urethra, but it restricts urethral descent during a pressure impulse caused by coughing or straining, and thus maintains continence.

Urinary frequency

A 55 year old woman attending your gynaecology clinic describes a 2 year history of 'running to the toilet all the time'. On further questioning she tells you that she passes urine 14 times per day and three times at night. On many of these occasions she does not reach the toilet before wetting herself.

What is the most likely diagnosis and what further questions might give information to support this diagnosis?

The most likely diagnosis is detrusor instability or urge incontinence. Other questions to ask are: 'Do you feel you pass a reasonable volume of urine each time you go to the toilet?', 'Do you feel you have emptied your bladder completely?' and 'Do you suffer from dribbling after urination?' Women with detrusor instability frequently describe passing small volumes of urine, the sensation of incomplete emptying and dribbling on standing after micturition. You should also determine if there is anything that makes it worse, whether she knows where all the toilets are when she goes shopping, and whether she feels the urge to go to the toilet as soon as she puts the key in the door when she gets home. Common precipitating factors for urgency are running water, cold and drinking fluids. These women often talk about going to the toilet 'just in case' and social outings are dominated by finding public toilets.

Establishing the degree of social inconvenience is an important aspect of the history.

Once the diagnosis of detrusor instability is suspected, what other information may be relevant?

It is important to establish whether the woman is postmenopausal and, if so, whether she is taking hormone replacement therapy, as oestrogen deficiency is often associated with symptoms of urge incontinence. One should also determine the pattern and type of fluid intake, as excessive volumes of fluid, large amounts of caffeine, and drinking before bedtime or during the night may all precipitate frequency and urgency. Medical and drug histories are important, as poorly controlled diabetes and diuretic tablets may mimic the symptoms of detrusor instability. Other salient features in the past medical history may be nocturnal enuresis as a child, previous pelvic surgery and any neurological symptoms.

What particular features would you look for on examination?

There may be atrophic changes of the vulva and vagina, but there should be no leaking of urine on coughing. It is important to look for uterovaginal prolapse, but isolated detrusor instability is not often associated with prolapse. Bimanual examination is typically normal. A neurogenic bladder should be excluded by testing for perineal sensation and the anal reflex, and a normal plantar response.

What simple investigations would you initiate?

Urinalysis should be performed for evidence of infection or haematuria, which might indicate the presence of bladder pathology. When this is positive, a midstream sample of urine should be sent for microscopy and culture. Urinary tract infection should be treated and persistent haematuria should be further investigated.

An ultrasound scan of the bladder post-micturition is a simple and non-invasive way of confirming complete emptying of the bladder.

A most useful exercise is to get the patient to keep a frequency and volume diary of her micturition. This will generally confirm the small-volume, frequent voiding pattern typical of detrusor instability, but will also help to detect patients who are drinking excessive volumes of fluid without realising it.

How would you manage this patient with detrusor instability?

A good starting point is to analyse the frequency and volume chart. This will demonstrate the nature and severity of the problem. If the total volume voided is very large and the volume of each void is good, volume restriction may be all that is needed. Caffeine is a diuretic and also irritates the bladder, so high caffeine intake should be addressed.

The keystone of management of the woman with detrusor instability is to bring about behavioural change. This is commonly achieved through a process called bladder drill, which is best performed in conjunction with pelvic floor exercises. The aims of bladder drill are to decrease the frequency of micturition and increase the volume of the urinary voids. The best way to attain this is by timed voiding. The idea is to start with a voiding interval that can be comfortably achieved without incontinence. The time interval is then slowly increased at the patient's own pace, so that the bladder gradually becomes accustomed to holding larger volumes. A good target is 3–4-hourly voids with volumes of 300 ml or more. Good pelvic floor tone assists this process by enabling the woman to reach the toilet in time, and sometimes by inhibiting urgency per se. This is often performed on an outpatient basis with the support of a physiotherapist or continence advisor, but in resistant cases a short inpatient stay with constant supervision may be helpful.

Additional help may be provided by either systemic or local oestrogen replacement therapy in the postmenopausal woman, and anticholinergic drugs. A common side-effect of anticholinergic drugs is a dry mouth, and in the past this led to high levels of non-compliance. A number of newer preparations in which this side-effect has been minimized are now available.

What further measures would you consider if there is no response to the conservative management outlined above?

Urodynamic studies should be performed to demonstrate detrusor instability definitively and to exclude other potential problems, such as a neurogenic bladder. These studies involve simultaneous measurement of the intra-abdominal and intravesical pressures by pressure transduction catheters placed in the vagina or rectum and the bladder. The pressure exerted by detrusor muscle tone is calculated by subtracting the intra-abdominal pressure (vaginal/rectal) from the intravesical pressure. These pressures are recorded while filling the bladder by transurethral infusion of saline or glycine. The volume at which there is first a desire to void and the maximum volume tolerated are recorded. The response to manoeuvres such as coughing or heel bouncing is assessed. Flow rates during micturition and the residual volume after voiding are also measured. Detrusor instability is demonstrated by involuntary elevation of the intravesical pressure and detrusor pressure without an increase in intra-abdominal pressure. Genuine stress incontinence is said to be present when the patient leaks on coughing without a detrusor contraction.

Cystoscopy should also be performed to exclude intravesical pathology, such as interstitial cystitis, transitional cell carcinoma and bladder stones.

A number of potential treatments are currently being investigated, one of which is sacral nerve stimulation. Detrusor contractions are inhibited by stimulation of the sacral nerve by a variety of different methods.

In the most resistant and debilitating cases, radical surgical intervention, such as clam cystoplasty or total cystectomy and ileal conduit, may be considered.

Prolapse

A 60 year old woman presents with a 6 month history of a 'feeling of something coming down'. There are no associated bladder symptoms. She describes no abnormal bleeding and her cervical smears to date have all been normal. The most likely diagnosis is uterovaginal prolapse.

Describe the different forms of female genital prolapse.

Vaginal wall prolapse is described according to the region of the vaginal wall that is deficient. Thus prolapse of the urethra is called a urethocele, prolapse of the bladder a cystocele, prolapse of the small intestine in the posterior fornix an enterocele and prolapse of the rectum a rectocele. If a hysterectomy has been performed, the vaginal vault may become prolapsed. When the uterus is in situ, the uterus and cervix may prolapse. The extent of uterine prolapse is often described in terms of three degrees: first degree is descent within the vagina; second degree is where the cervix reaches the introitus; and third degree is where the uterine body descends beyond the introitus (Fig. 22.1).

What factors contribute to uterovaginal prolapse?

Uterovaginal prolapse is caused by stretching and subsequent weakness of the supporting ligaments and fascia. The predominant cause is vaginal childbirth, and prolapse is thought to be most common in women of high parity who have had big babies and prolonged labours. Recurrent elevation of intra-abdominal pressure due to obesity, chronic cough or constipation may exacerbate the problem. Loss of tissue elasticity secondary to oestrogen deficiency may also contribute after the menopause. In rare instances prolapse may be congenital and occur at a young age in a nulliparous woman.

On examination you find atrophic changes of the vulva, vagina and cervix, and second degree uterine prolapse, with perineal deficiency and a cystocele and rectocele. What additional information do you want to elicit on pelvic examination?

A bimanual examination should be performed to assess the size and mobility of the uterus, and the presence of any adnexal masses, as these findings may influence surgical management.

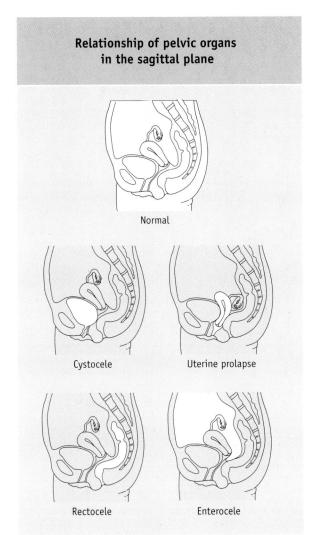

Relationship of pelvic organs in the sagittal plane

Normal

Cystocele

Uterine prolapse

Rectocele

Enterocele

Fig. 22.1 *Relationship of pelvic organs in the sagittal plane. Anticlockwise from top: sagittal view of pelvic organs; middle left: bladder bulging into vagina to produce a cystocele; bottom left: rectum bulging into vagina to produce a rectocele; bottom right: peritoneal sac bulging into vagina to produce an enterocele; middle right: uterine descent into the vagina.*

Is there a role for conservative management, and what approach might this take?

Definitive management of uterovaginal prolapse is surgery to restore normal anatomical relationships. However, not all patients will wish to undergo surgery and some will not be fit for anaesthesia. These women may benefit from the insertion of a ring pessary, which supports the uterus and anterior vaginal wall by resting on the upper border of the symphysis pubis. It is important to fit the correct size of ring: too small a ring may be expelled on straining; too large a ring may cause discomfort and difficulty passing urine. Regular topical oestrogen therapy is required in a post-menopausal woman to prevent erosion of the ring through the vaginal epithelium. The ring should be changed every 4–6 months to allow inspection of the vaginal mucosa and to reduce the risk of infection. Conservative management may also ameliorate symptoms while the patient is awaiting surgery. Pelvic floor exercises are unlikely to reduce prolapse, but when performed after surgery they may help to prevent recurrence.

What surgical intervention might be appropriate in this case?

The most common procedure in this situation would be vaginal hysterectomy to remove the prolapsing uterus and cervix, combined with repair of the cystocele and rectocele. The deficient perineum can also be corrected by extending the posterior repair to include a perineorrhaphy.

Another surgical procedure that may be employed is a sacrospinous colpopexy. This involves attaching the cervix to the sacrospinous ligament, usually on one side (most commonly the right). The sacrospinous ligament is accessed via the posterior vaginal wall and the ischiorectal fossa. The incision in the posterior vaginal wall can be incorporated into a posterior repair. The advantages of this procedure are that it restores the primary support of the uterus, conserves the uterus, and preserves the length of the vagina.

Vaginal hysterectomy with sacrospinous fixation of the vaginal vault combines the main features of both of these operations.

What structures are clamped, cut and tied when performing a vaginal hysterectomy?

The first clamp includes the uterosacral and transverse cervical ligaments. Working upwards, the next clamp occludes the uterine arteries, and the final clamp divides the fallopian tubes, round ligaments, broad ligaments and ovarian ligaments.

When repairing the posterior vaginal wall, how can a rectocele be distinguished from an enterocele?

This distinction can be difficult to make on direct inspection of the posterior wall. A simple way of demonstrating the extent of a rectocele is to pass a finger into the rectum and press it forwards. The finger will enter and delineate the bulge of the rectocele. Any swelling above this is due to an enterocele. Unlike a rectocele, an enterocele is covered with a sac of peritoneum, which should be reduced when repairing it.

Postmenopausal bleeding

A 55 year old woman presents with a history of vaginal bleeding on two occasions over the past 3 months.

What are the salient points that you should elucidate on history?

The first thing to establish is that the woman is truly menopausal. The menopause is considered to have occurred when, in a woman of climacteric age, there have been no menses for 6 months or more.

The next thing is to determine the details of the presenting symptom, such as when the bleeding occurred, how heavy it was, whether it was fresh or old blood, how long it lasted and whether there were any precipitating factors. Heavy, fresh bleeding that recurs or is prolonged suggests a more sinister aetiology. Another important question is whether the woman is taking hormone replacement therapy or any other drug, such as tamoxifen or warfarin, which may be associated with abnormal uterine bleeding. The cervical screening history should be documented, as the bleeding may be cervical in origin.

Other relevant points in the history are factors that are associated with an increased risk of endometrial carcinoma, such as nulliparity, obesity, diabetes and other conditions, such as polycystic ovary syndrome, that are linked with chronic anovulation and unopposed oestrogen stimulation of the endometrium.

What are the potential causes of postmenopausal bleeding?

The most important conditions to exclude are carcinomas of the genital tract. The most common to present with postmenopausal bleeding is endometrial carcinoma, but cervical, vaginal, urethral and vulval carcinomas may also present in this way. Other causes are best categorized in terms of their anatomical site. Vulval causes include excoriation due to itch and ulceration, which may be due to conditions such as genital herpes and Behçet disease. A urethral caruncle may present as postmenopausal bleeding. Vaginal causes include atrophic vaginitis and vaginal tears. Polyps and chronic inflammation may cause bleeding from the cervix. Endometrial polyps and endometrial hyperplasia are common intrauterine causes.

What examination and investigations would you instigate?

A brief general examination is appropriate in a patient who may require an anaesthetic for a surgical procedure. The abdomen should be palpated to exclude a mass arising from the pelvis. A full pelvic examination should then be performed. The vulva, vagina and cervix are inspected for lesions described above. It may be appropriate to take a cervical smear if routine screening is due or if the appearance is in any way suspicious. A bimanual examination will reveal the size, position and mobility of the uterus, and the presence of any adnexal mass.

A helpful investigation is transvaginal ultrasonography of the uterus, looking specifically at the endometrium. Uniformly thickened endometrium may indicate hyperplasia or malignancy, and an area of localized thickening may represent a polyp. An outpatient endometrial biopsy is useful to improve the accuracy of diagnosis, but if the appearance of the endometrium on ultrasound is suspicious, a hysteroscopy and directed biopsy may be indicated.

Hysteroscopy has commonly been performed as a day-surgery procedure but there is an increasing trend towards outpatient hysteroscopy, as examination using a thin modern hysteroscope is generally well tolerated. An operating channel in the sheath of the hysteroscope allows directed biopsies to be taken.

Transvaginal ultrasonography shows the endometrium to be 12 mm thick and you proceed to hysteroscopy and directed biopsy. Histopathology reveals simple hyperplasia with no atypia. How would you manage this patient?

If left untreated, simple hyperplasia may rarely become hyperplasia with atypia, which may be considered as a precursor to endometrial carcinoma. However, simple hyperplasia will usually revert to normal under the influence of progestogen therapy. Progestogen is commonly given in the form of continuous oral therapy, but an alternative approach is to insert a progestogen releasing intrauterine system. The response to progestogen therapy can be monitored by a follow-up endometrial biopsy after a few months.

Recurrent miscarriages

A 34 year old women presents to your gynaecology clinic with a history of three miscarriages; she wants to know if there is a treatable cause.

What information in her history may help you establish if there is a cause?

Recurrent miscarriage is defined as three or more consecutive pregnancy losses and is thought to affect 1% of all women. As miscarriage is such a common event (approximately 1 in 5 pregnancies), statistical probability alone will dictate that some women will have three or more consecutive miscarriages by pure misfortune. In the majority of cases, no underlying cause can be found, but for an important minority, investigation will reveal a likely explanation.

It is important to establish when the miscarriages occurred, i.e. in the first or second trimester. Second trimester miscarriage may be due to cervical incompetence, a condition that presents with silent dilatation of the cervix, typically at 19–20 weeks gestation. Cervical incompetence is often overdiagnosed and treatment by vaginally placed cervical cerclage has been shown to be ineffective in terms of fetal survival in a RCOG/MRC (Royal College of Obstetricians and Gynaecologists/Medical Research Council) trial. There is interest in transabdominal cervical cerclage both preconceptually and during pregnancy. Reports of pregnancy outcome have been promising, but there is little evidence from randomized controlled trials to support this management.

Other important information relates to the patient and her partner's genetic history. They should be asked whether any of their close relatives have had similar difficulties with reproduction and whether they are aware of any genetic conditions running in their families. The general medical well-being of the couple should be established, and in particular any conditions suffered by the woman. A number of chronic diseases may result in recurrent miscarriage; for example, poorly controlled diabetes and systemic lupus erythematosus. Medications may also be important. An example is methotrexate, used for the management of rheumatoid arthritis; this is a cytotoxic drug and may cause miscarriage if conception occurs while the woman is taking it.

What investigations will you instigate?

Despite the low overall yield, there are a few key investigations that enable us to give meaningful counselling or to initiate treatment that has a reasonable chance of securing a successful pregnancy outcome. Between 3 and 5% of couples with recurrent miscarriage will have a genetic cause, such as a balanced reciprocal or a robertsonian translocation. It is therefore important to check the karyotype of both partners. If an abnormality is detected, the couple should be referred for genetic counselling. This should include the likelihood of the underlying genetic abnormality resulting in miscarriage or fetal abnormality in a given pregnancy, the possible need for other family members to be screened, and whether pregnancy outcome might be improved by embryo selection or prenatal diagnosis.

The antiphospholipid syndrome is another important cause of recurring pregnancy loss. It can be diagnosed by the presence of either anticardiolipin antibodies (of either the IgG or IgM class) or lupus anticoagulant. Approximately 15% of women with recurrent miscarriage will have these antibodies, in comparison to < 1% of a low-risk population. Due to the fact that there may be temporary changes in these antibody levels, it is recommended that they be tested for on two occasions 6 weeks apart (when the woman is not pregnant), and tests only be considered affirmative if the same antibody is positive on both occasions. Increasingly, heritable thrombophilia is also recognized to be associated with recurrent and late miscarriage. The mechanism may be similar to the antiphospholipid antibody syndrome, with thrombotic damage to the placenta. It may therefore be useful to ask about any family history of thrombosis and consider performing a thrombophilia screen.

Another investigation that may be helpful is a transvaginal ultrasound scan to look at ovarian and uterine morphology. Structural abnormalities of the uterus are often blamed for recurrent pregnancy loss, despite many reports of normal pregnancies in women with uterine septae. In the majority of cases, surgery is likely to be of little benefit. Women who underwent open procedures in the past had a high subsequent rate of infertility. Hysteroscopic surgery may be more successful but has not yet been fully evaluated. There are many endocrine tests that were previously considered important when investigating recurrent pregnancy loss. These included thyroid function tests and HbA1c. However, evidence now available shows that, unless the patient has clinical manifestations of thyroid disease or diabetes, these investigations are unnecessary.

The woman is found to have consistently elevated IgG anticardiolipin levels. What treatment would you suggest?

The combination of low-dose aspirin (75 mg) and heparin (usually low molecular weight heparin is used, e.g. 40 mg enoxaparin daily is employed in this situation. Low molecular weight heparins are preferable as they have a substantially lower risk of side-effects, particularly heparin-induced thrombocytopenia and osteoporosis, compared with unfractionated heparin. This therapy is started on diagnosis of pregnancy. Randomised trials have shown this treatment to reduce significantly the risk of miscarriage. It is continued at least until the second trimester. There is merit in continuing it further, in view of the association between antiphospholipid antibodies and late pregnancy loss, as well as pre-eclampsia and intrauterine growth restriction (IUGR), although there is no evidence from controlled trials that these late pregnancy complications will be reduced by this treatment. As these antibodies also place the woman at risk of venous thrombosis, heparin therapy will provide thromboprophylaxis as well.

Contraception

An 18 year old presents to a family planning clinic, requesting contraception.

What are the important points of the history that you should ascertain?

A sexual history is imperative in order to establish the reason for her request, and her risk status for pregnancy and sexually transmitted infection. A good starting point may be the open-ended question, 'Why are you seeking contraception?' The answer may give you a framework for other, more specific questions. You should try to establish whether the young woman is already sexually active or considering becoming so; whether she is in a stable relationship or engaging in casual sex; and what (if any) contraception she has already been using.

What methods of contraception are available, and how effective are they (Fig. 25.1)?

Many different types of contraception are available; they can be divided into a number of categories, namely natural methods, barrier methods, chemical methods, hormonal methods, intra-uterine contraceptive devices and systems (IUCD/IUS), and sterilization. The efficacy of a contraceptive method is defined per 100 woman-years. This can be a confusing concept, but the following two ways of interpreting it may make it more meaningful. If 100 women used the method of contraception for 1 year, the rate given is the number of those women who might conceive a pregnancy within that year. Alternatively, if the rate given is divided into 100, it will give the number of years of using the method regularly in which a pregnancy is likely to occur, i.e. a rate of 5 per 100 woman-years means that, for a given individual, it is likely that one pregnancy will occur within 20 years of regular use (as $100 \div 5 = 20$).

Natural methods of contraception include coitus interruptus and fertility awareness. Both have an efficacy ranging from 6–20 per 100 woman-years. Coitus interruptus is a particularly poor method from the woman's perspective, as she has virtually no control over the situation. The effectiveness of fertility awareness can be greatly improved by using the Billing method to assess cervical mucus, or by using a cycle monitoring device such as Persona®.

The most commonly used barrier method is the male condom. Other barrier methods include the female condom, diaphragms, cervical caps and the contraceptive sponge, all of which are inserted into the vagina by the woman and aim to occlude the cervical os. Regarding their efficacy, the failure rates are as shown in Fig. 25.1, overleaf. All of these failure rates are dependent on the experience and motivation of the user, with older couples tending to have a lower failure rate than their

Lowest expected and typical pregnancy rates for commonly used contraceptive methods

Method	Lowest expected pregnancy rate (%)	Typical pregnancy rate (%)
Combined oral contraceptive	0.10	3.00
Depot progestogen	0.30	0.30
Progestogen implant	0.04	0.20
Intrauterine contraceptive device	<0.10	3.00
Condoms	2.00	12.00
Cap	6.00	18.00
Female sterilization	0.20	0.40
Male sterilization	0.10	0.15
Natural family planning	1–9	20.00

Fig. 25.1 Lowest expected and typical pregnancy rates for commonly used contraceptive methods.

younger counterparts.

Hormonal methods of contraception vary in the type of hormones used and the method of delivery (Fig. 25.2). Oral preparations are the combined oral contraceptive pill, which contains both oestrogen and progestogen, and the progestogen-only pill. Progestogen-only contraception can also be delivered by subcutaneous depot injection (Depo-

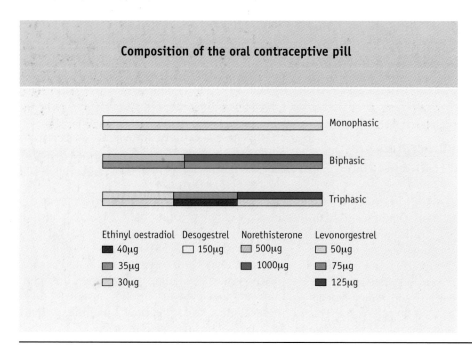

Composition of the oral contraceptive pill

Monophasic

Biphasic

Triphasic

Ethinyl oestradiol
- 40µg
- 35µg
- 30µg

Desogestrel
- 150µg

Norethisterone
- 500µg
- 1000µg

Levonorgestrel
- 50µg
- 75µg
- 125µg

Fig. 25.2 The combined oral contraceptive pill is a combination of synthetic oestrogen and synthetic progestogen.

Provera®), subcutaneous implant (Implanon®), and the levonorgestrel-releasing intrauterine system (Mirena®). The respective failure rates of these methods are 0.2–3 per 100 woman-years for the combined oral contraceptive pill, 0.3–4 per 100 woman-years for the progestogen-only pill, <1 per 100 woman-years for Depo-Provera, <1 per 100 woman-years for Implanon, and <0.5 per 100 woman-years for Mirena.

Modern intrauterine devices all contain copper to increase their efficacy, which ranges from 0.3 to 1 per 100 woman-years.

Sterilization is a popular method of contraception in later reproductive years, but is clearly not appropriate for this patient.

What would be important considerations in deciding the best form of contraception for this 18 year old woman?

Important considerations are her age, her nulliparity, the likelihood of exposure to more than one partner (either through casual encounters or serial monogamy), and her motivation to use contraception reliably.

She has heard the expression 'double Dutch' and asks you what this means.

The expression double Dutch refers to taking the oral contraceptive pill and also using condoms. This combination was popularized in Holland, as a means of protecting against sexually transmitted infections as well as preventing pregnancy. It was particularly aimed at younger women, who have a higher risk of sexually transmitted infections and are also more fertile than older women.

She enquires about an IUCD. How would you counsel her about this form of contraception?

The IUCD is a small device, generally made from a combination of plastic and copper. The presence of a foreign body within the uterus induces an inflammatory response, which, along with the copper ions, acts by impeding sperm transport and fertilization of the oocyte. These effects also impair implantation of the blastocyst, which is a useful back-up mechanism in general use, and is the main mechanism of action when an IUCD is used for emergency contraception.

The IUCD is a highly effective form of contraception that requires minimal input from the user. General disadvantages are an association with heavier, more painful periods, incomplete protection against ectopic pregnancy, complications of fitting the device, and the risk of expulsion. Particular disadvantages for the young woman relate to the fact that she is at higher risk of sexually transmitted infections. Such infections are more likely to be worsened by the insertion or presence of an IUCD and may thus result in tubal occlusion and infertility. Thus it is not usually the first-choice contraceptive for a young woman.

Endometriosis

A 31 year old woman presents to your gynaecology clinic with a 12 month history of pelvic pain and dyspareunia.

What is your differential diagnosis and what information obtained from the history will help you to distinguish between them.

The differential diagnosis includes endometriosis, pelvic inflammatory disease (PID), irritable bowel syndrome and psychosexual causes.

Endometriosis is a potential cause of these symptoms. Associated features may include pre-menstrual pelvic pain, which tends to improve when the period comes. Heavy painful periods are often associated. Very occasionally unusual symptoms, such as rectal bleeding or haematuria only at the time of menstruation, may suggest ectopic endometriosis in the rectum or bladder.

PID is usually an acute problem associated with vaginal discharge and systemic symptoms such as pyrexia and nausea. The fact that in this case the symptoms have been present for 12 months makes it an unlikely cause. PID can be chronic and enquiry regarding the presence of a vaginal discharge, a past history of PID or a partner with a history of sexually transmitted disease is important.

Irritable bowel syndrome commonly presents with pelvic pain, although dyspareunia would be an uncommon complaint with this condition. Other associated symptoms, such as constipation, diarrhoea and abdominal bloating, are generally related to the bowel.

Other more unusual causes may be the presence of a pelvic mass, either fibroid uterus or an ovarian cyst, and the patient may have noticed a lump in her abdomen and/or associated pressure symptoms on the bowel or bladder. A change in menstrual pattern, such as heavier bleeding, may point towards the fibroid uterus; erratic or stopped may suggest an ovarian cyst.

A pychosexual cause for the problem should be considered if no other cause is found on investigation.

The patient reports that she gets pelvic pain a week before her period and that her periods have become increasingly painful and heavy. You suspect endometriosis is the likely diagnosis. What investigations will you instigate now to confirm your diagnosis?

The gold standard investigation for the diagnosis of this condition is still a laparoscopy to look directly into the pelvis for evidence of endometriosis.

A pelvic ultrasound may be helpful, especially to detect the presence of endometriomas, ovarian cysts caused by endometriosis involving the ovaries. A raised CA 125 level may be detected by taking a blood sample from the patient. This is not very sensitive or specific but may be useful in the monitoring of treatment of already diagnosed endometriosis.

What is endometriosis, and what does it look like at laparoscopy? How can you be certain that what you see actually is endometriosis?

Endometriosis is the presence of tissue that is histologically similar to endometrium at sites outside the uterus. It is commonly found on the ovary and on the pelvic peritoneum, especially the uterosacral ligaments, broad ligament, uterovesical peritoneum and the pouch of Douglas (Fig. 26.1). When it is found within the myometrium it is termed adenomyosis. The classic symptoms of endometriosis are pelvic pain, deep dyspareunia and dysmenorrhoea. It is considered to arise as a consequence of the dissemination and implantation of endometrium at ectopic sites by retrograde menstruation along the fallopian tubes, or possibly spread through the blood vessels or lymphatics. Endometriosis is an oestrogen-dependent condition occuring only in women during their reproductive years, and symptoms are often cyclical. It often resolves during pregnancy and after the menopause.

The appearance of endometriosis can vary considerably at laparoscopy (Fig. 26.2). Endometriosis may be red, black or brown. Lesions may appear nodular or vesicular or may look like powder burns. The only way to be absolutely certain of your diagnosis is to perform a biopsy to confirm histologically that endometriosis is present.

How can you treat endometriosis?

Treatment of endometriosis is divided into medical management and surgical management.

Medical management may simply be prescription of analgesics, such as non-steroidal anti-inflammatory drugs. Other medical therapy tends to be the use of hormonal preparations. The aim

Distribution of endometriosis in the pelvis

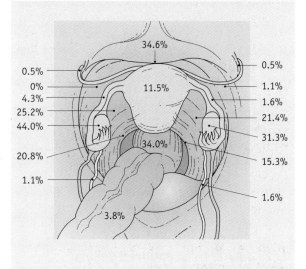

Fig. 26.1 Distribution of endometriosis in the pelvis illustrating the frequency for various anatomical sites as determined in a laparoscopic study. (From the American College of Obstetricians and Gynecologists 1986 Obstetrics and Gynecology 67: 335–338, with permission.)

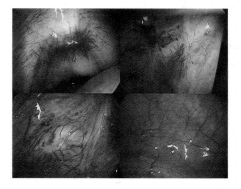

Fig. 26.2 Endometriosis is associated with many different visual appearances. One of the features of the disease is angiogenesis. Top left: active endometriosis with angiogenesis between the uterosacral ligaments. Top right: classic blue-black lesions. Bottom left: no pigmentation; the blue-black colour results from the deposition of haemosiderin. Bottom right: normal peritoneum for comparison.

of hormonal treatment is to induce atrophy in the endometriosis. There are various medications available to the treating doctor; these include the combined oral contraceptive pill, oral progestogens, danazol and GnRH agonists. All these medications have similar efficacy in controlling the pain and causing atrophy of the endometriosis. Unfortunately, there is a significant recurrence rate after cessation of the treatment, and long-term therapy can be difficult due to side-affects related to the medication.

Surgical treatment involves ablation of the endometriosis. This is usually performed laparoscopically. It can be very successful in many women. Those in whom it fails tend to have either incomplete ablation of the disease or a recurrence of it. Symptomatic relief may be improved by following surgical treatment with GnRH agonists.

How do you treat endometriomas?

The treatment of endometriomas usually involves surgical excision and or drainage. This can be performed as a laparoscopic or an open procedure. Medical treatment is relatively ineffective for endometriomas.

Endometriosis is often associated with infertility. How does it cause infertility and what is the most effective treatment?

Endometriosis can cause infertility by directly damaging the pelvic organs, such as the fallopian tubes or the ovaries. It may also cause infertility indirectly by affecting the gametes and fertilization process with the production of local substances (although IVF results for women with endometriosis are fairly good). The most effective treatment for endometriosis-related infertility appears, from the literature, to be surgical. Surgical treatment results in higher pregnancy rates post-treatment; however, surgery can be avoided by using IVF techniques that have good success rates in women with this condition.

SECTION 3

Pregnancy problems

Age over 35 years

A 40 year old primigravid statistician presents at 10 weeks gestation. She is aware that the incidence of Down syndrome is increased with increasing maternal age and wishes to discuss her options.

What is her risk of having a baby with a chromosomal abnormality, based on age alone?

The incidence of chromosomal abnormality based on age alone depends on gestation (higher with earlier gestation as chromosomally abnormal fetuses are more likely to miscarry), previously affected pregnancies and known parental chromosomal problems. A useful approximate rule, however, is:

Maternal age (years)	Incidence of chromosomal abnormality (approximate)
20	1:2000
30	1:1000
35	1:350
40	1:100
45	1:40

The majority of these will be Down syndrome, but a small proportion may be Edwards (trisomy 18), Patau (trisomy 13), other autosomal trisomies and triploidy.

Are her risks of structural abnormality (e.g. spina bifida) also age related?

The incidence of these does not increase with increased maternal age. If the mother does want to be screened for these abnormalities they are best identified with an ultrasound scan, and many clinicians advocate that all mothers should be offered at least one detailed ultrasound at around 18–20 weeks or earlier. This has the advantage that termination can be offered in cases of previously unsuspected major or lethal anomalies (e.g. spina bifida, renal agenesis), and it also allows planned deliveries in those conditions that may require early neonatal intervention (e.g. gastroschisis, transposition of the great arteries).

Many structural problems, however, are not identified by scanning (it is likely that < 50% of cardiac defects are recognized) and the false reassurance provided by this scan may become a source of parental resentment. Furthermore, some other problem may be uncovered; for example, one of the 'soft markers' (see below), the natural history of which is uncertain. This may generate unnecessary anxiety and increase the number of invasive diagnostic procedures (and thereby the loss rate) in otherwise normal pregnancies.

What are the features of Down syndrome?

Although walking, language and self-care skills are usually attained, independence is rare. There is mental retardation (with a mean IQ around 50) and an association with congenital heart disease (particularly atrioventricular canal defects, ventricular septal defect, patent ductus arteriosus, atrial septal defect primum and Fallot's tetralogy). Gastrointestinal atresias are common, and there is early dementia, with similarities to Alzheimer disease. Twenty per cent of those affected die before the age of 1 year; 45% reach 60 years of age.

What are her options when considering the risk of Down syndrome?

- No tests
- Screening tests with either:
  - ultrasound measurement of the nuchal translucency between 11 and 14 weeks, ± chorionic villus sampling if screen positive
  - serum alpha-fetoprotein, human chorionic gonadotrophin (± unconjugated estriol) at 15 + weeks, ± amniocentesis if screen positive
- Diagnostic tests without screening:
  - chorionic villus sampling
  - amniocentesis at 15 weeks gestation.

What are the pros and cons of each?

The 'no test' option speaks for itself. This patient has an age-related risk of around 1:100 or, more

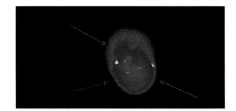

Fig. 27.1   *Fluorescence in situ hybridization (FISH).*

reassuringly, there will be a 99% chance that the baby will not have Down syndrome.

The screening process attempts to provide an individualized risk for Down syndrome. One way is to measure maternal serum alpha-fetoprotein and human chorionic gonadotrophin (± unconjugated oestriol levels) at 15 + weeks gestation. By correcting these for maternal weight and adjusting the results for maternal age, some 60% of cases can be picked up by recalling approximately 4% of the screened population for amniocentesis. With amniocentesis, a needle is inserted into the uterus transabdominally to remove 10–15 ml of amniotic fluid. Karyotype results are usually available within 3 weeks, but fluorescence in situ hybridization (FISH) and polymerase chain reaction (PCR) techniques may be used to exclude the more common aneuploidies within 72 h (Fig. 27.1). The disadvantage with amniocentesis, however, is that it carries a miscarriage rate of 0.5–1%.

It is also possible to screen by measuring the fetal nuchal thickness on first trimester ultrasound (Fig. 27.2). Sensitivities of over 80% have been quoted for the detection of Down syndrome, particularly if combined with additional serum

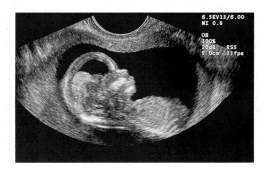

Fig. 27.2   *Nuchal translucency.*

markers. Chorionic villus sampling, in which a needle is used to biopsy the placenta, is required as the diagnostic test (amniocentesis should not be carried out before 15 weeks) and this probably carries a higher miscarriage rate (around 2–3%). Results are usually available within 48 h. Diagnosis at these earlier gestations allows the option of surgical termination which, although perhaps simpler, may not necessarily be psychologically advantageous. Increased nuchal translucency is also a marker for structural defects (4% of those > 3 mm), particularly cardiac, diaphragmatic hernia, renal, abdominal wall and other more rare abnormalities.

Opting directly for either amniocentesis or chorionic villus sampling has the advantage of accurate diagnosis but the disadvantage of miscarriage risks.

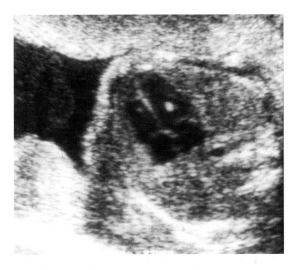

Fig. 27.4   *A left ventricular echogenic focus.*

She has heard about the use of soft markers. What are they?

These are structural features found on ultrasound, which in themselves are not a problem but which may be pointers to aneuploidy. The more common are choroid plexus cysts (Fig. 27.3), calcification of the cardiac papillary muscle ('echogenic foci', Fig. 27.4), renal pelvic dilatation (Fig. 27.5), mild cerebral ventricular dilatation and echogenic

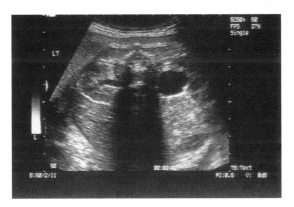

Fig. 27.5   *The left renal pelvis, is normal at 3 mm, but the right side is significantly dilated at 12 mm.*

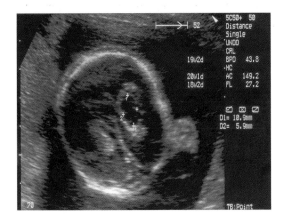

Fig. 27.3   *An isolated choroid plexus cyst.*

bowel. They are found in approximately 5% of all pregnancies in the second trimester and are the cause of much parental anxiety. Assignment of risk for aneuploidy is fraught with difficulty as adequate data from low-risk pregnancies are limited. If isolated, the risk of chromosomal problems is low. If more than one is found, or if there are any other structural defects, the risk is very much higher. They should not be relied upon as a screening test for chromosomal abnormalities — the majority of fetuses with Down syndrome look normal on ultrasound scan.

As she is a statistician, she wishes to use statistics to decide what is best. She asks you about what, statistically, is the right answer for her?

While it is easy to generalize with population-based statistics, she must make up her own mind what is right for her, based on her views about the risk, her feelings about prenatal testing and her feelings about Down syndrome itself (some couples would not wish to have a termination). It will also depend on her views about coping with the uncertainties of screening tests versus the specifics of diagnostic tests. Mathematics alone cannot be used to find the answer.

It is important to note that the pick-up rate of these screening tests (sensitivity) is higher in older women, but the chance of being recalled with an elevated risk is also higher (35% if under 25 years, > 90% if over 40 years). It is therefore not necessary or appropriate to advise women over the age of 35 years to have an amniocentesis but they should be aware that their chance of recall is significantly increased.

After considering the ethical questions associated with prenatal diagnosis, she opts not to take any test. In the light of the fact that she is 40 years of age, what other obstetric factors would you wish to consider?

There is a slightly increased risk of both fetal and maternal problems with increasing maternal age, particularly preterm labour, pre-eclampsia and venous thromboembolic disease. The incidence of intrauterine death, instrumental delivery and caesarean section is also slightly higher in this age group. It may be appropriate to discuss induction, or some form of monitoring, as term approaches and to consider postnatal thromboembolic prophylaxis.

Previous birth of a baby with spina bifida

A 24 year old para 0+1 was found 2 years previously to have an elevated alpha-fetoprotein level at 16 weeks gestation and a subsequent scan showed that the baby had spina bifida. She elected for termination of pregnancy.

She was advised to take folic acid in her next pregnancy. Why?

There is very good evidence that folic acid taken from before conception reduces the recurrence risk of neural tube defects in those who have had a previously affected child. The usual dose is 400 μg per day but some obstetricians prescribe 5 mg tablets. There is no apparent risk from folic acid supplements.

She is aware that her risk of neural tube defect recurrence is around 5%. What are neural tube defects?

The neural tube is formed from the closing of the neural folds, with both anterior and posterior neuropores closed by 6 weeks gestation (Fig. 28.1). Failure of closure of the anterior neuropore results in anencephaly or an encephalocele, and failure of posterior closure in spina bifida.

Anencephaly

The skull vault and cerebral cortex are absent. The infant is either stillborn or, if liveborn, will usually die shortly after birth (although some may survive for several days).

Encephalocele

There is a bony defect in the cranial vault through which a dura mater sac (± brain tissue) protrudes. This may be occipital or frontal. Isolated meningoceles carry a good prognosis, whereas those with microcephaly secondary to brain herniation carry a very poor prognosis.

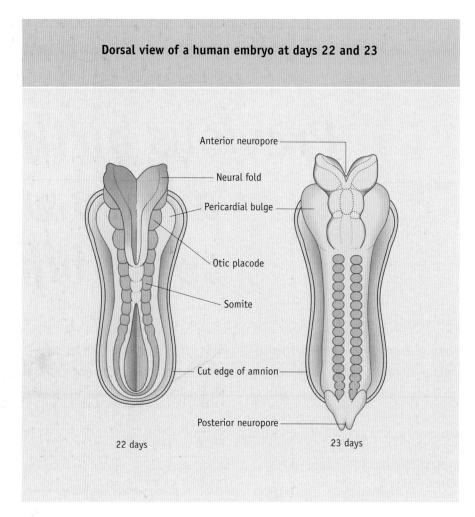

Dorsal view of a human embryo at days 22 and 23

Anterior neuropore

Neural fold

Pericardial bulge

Otic placode

Somite

Cut edge of amnion

Posterior neuropore

22 days

23 days

Fig. 28.1   Closure of the anterior and posterior neuropores.

Spina bifida (Fig. 28.2)

In a meningocele, dura and arachnoid mater bulge through the defect, whereas in a myelomeningocele, the cord itself is also exposed. Those with spinal meningoceles usually have normal lower limb neurology, and 20% have hydrocephalus. Those with myelomeningoceles usually have abnormal lower limb neurology and many have hydrocephalus. In addition to immobility and mental retardation there may be problems with urinary tract infections, bladder dysfunction, bowel dysfunction, and social and sexual isolation. Spina bifida and anencephaly make up more than 95% of neural tube defects. There is wide geographical variation in births, with a higher incidence in Scotland and Ireland (3:1000), and a lower incidence in England (2:1000), USA, Canada, Japan and Africa (< 1:1000). There is good evidence that the overall incidence has fallen over the past 15 years (independent of any screening programmes).

How would you screen for neural defects in this patient?

A scan should be arranged for 10–11 weeks to exclude anencephaly. Spina bifida can be excluded by scan at 17–18 weeks gestation.

fetuses with spina bifida and carries a much poorer prognosis than spina bifida alone. Markers for spina bifida (which are 99% sensitive) include blunting of the sinciput (lemon sign), a banana-shaped cerebellum (Arnold–Chiari malformation) and an absent cerebellum (Figs 28.4, 28.5).

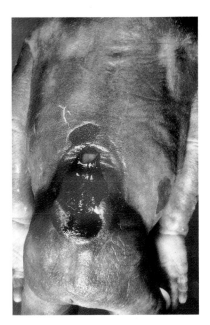

Fig. 28.2 *There is a large lumbosacral spina bifida. A termination of pregnancy was carried out at 19 weeks gestation.*

The spine can be viewed by ultrasound in three planes to assess the type and level of any deficit (Fig. 28.3). Hydrocephalus occurs in about 90% of

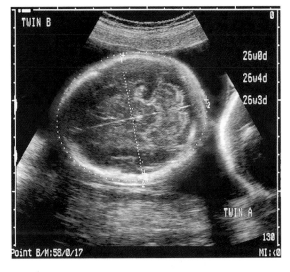

Fig. 28.4 *Normal cerebellum – this finding makes a neural tube defect very unlikely.*

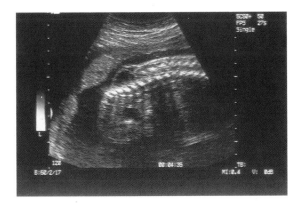

Fig. 28.3 *Sagittal view of a lumbar myelomeningocele.*

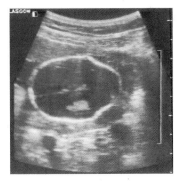

Fig. 28.5 *Lemon sign – there is blunting of the sinciput so that the head appears more pointed anteriorly.*

Essential hypertension

A 37 year old primigravida attends the antenatal clinic for booking at 9 weeks gestation. She tells you that she has a history of high blood pressure, which has been investigated by the physicians in the past with no cause found. Her blood pressure is usually controlled with atenolol 100 mg daily.

What risks does she face in pregnancy and how would you manage her care?

Chronic hypertension, usually essential hypertension, complicates between 1 and 2% of pregnancies. It is usually identified as a persistent elevation of blood pressure in the first or early second trimester and often the patient will have a past history of hypertension. In this case, the woman has already been investigated for underlying causes, such as renal and connective tissue disease, and thus the presumed diagnosis would be essential hypertension. If there is any doubt about this, the situation should be clarified by contact with the general practitioner or the treating physician because it is critical to exclude such problems, some of which may have significant implications for the pregnancy. With essential hypertension there is a significantly increased risk of IUGR and pre-eclampsia: regular assessment of fetal growth in the second half of pregnancy, with careful assessment for signs or symptoms of pre-eclampsia, must be instituted.

Can her atenolol therapy be withdrawn?

Women with essential hypertension generally show the same fall in blood pressure as occurs in normal pregnancy. Blood pressure starts to decline in the first trimester, reaching a nadir in mid-pregnancy, before slowly increasing in the third trimester to values compatible with those seen before pregnancy. Because of this, it is often possible to stop antihypertensive medication when the physiological fall in blood pressure occurs, although reinstitution of treatment is often required in the late part of the second or the third trimester. It is also important to consider the therapeutic agent. Chronic antihypertensive therapy, particularly with adrenoreceptor antagonists such as atenolol, are associated with reduced fetal growth. While initially this was considered to be a feature of adrenoceptor antagonists alone, recent data suggest that it may be the chronic reduction in blood pressure that is important, rather than a specific drug effect. Continuing treatment with antihypertensive agents will not reduce the risk of pre-eclampsia developing. Thus withdrawing antihypertensive medication may reduce the risk of IUGR. Some clinicians employ low-dose aspirin in an attempt to prevent such complications, although its benefits in this situation are unproven.

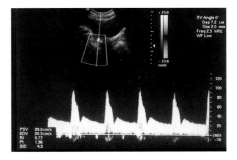

Fig. 29.1 *Uterine artery Doppler ultrasound examination showing notching.*

Are any tests available to predict whether she will develop pre-eclampsia or IUGR?

In view of the increased risk of pregnancy complications it may be of value to perform Doppler ultrasound assessment of the uterine arteries (Fig. 29.1). The presence of a persistent notching pattern at 22 weeks gestation, which is thought to reflect failure of the second wave of trophoblast invasion (a key feature of pre-eclampsia and IUGR), may be useful in helping to identify patients at increased risk. Should such a persistent notching pattern be present, consideration could be given to low-dose aspirin therapy at this time; alternatively, antioxidant vitamin supplements could be employed. A recent study has shown encouraging data where women with persistent notching were randomized to receive vitamin C and vitamin E supplements or placebo, with a more favourable outcome than those receiving these antioxidant vitamins. While encouraging, further information is required on the efficacy of such therapy, particularly in situations such as essential hypertension.

If her blood pressure rises in the third trimester, how do you know if this reflects her essential hypertension or the development of pre-eclampsia?

When blood pressure starts to increase in the late second and third trimester in the patient with essential hypertension, it can often be difficult to determine whether this is simply a physiological increase in blood pressure or the development of superimposed pregnancy-induced hypertension or pre-eclampsia. Increased plasma urate concentrations or the development of proteinuria are usually indicative of pre-eclampsia developing. Should antihypertensive therapy be required, agents such as atenolol, labetalol or methyldopa can be employed, with calcium channel blocking agents such as nifedipine being prescribed as second-line therapy.

Bleeding in early pregnancy

A 22 year old woman attends you with a 12 h history of vaginal bleeding accompanied by cramping lower abdominal pain. She has had 6 weeks amenorrhoea and tells you that she recently used a urinary pregnancy test from her local pharmacy; the test proved to be positive. She has had no previous pregnancies and was using no contraception.

What is the differential diagnosis?

The differential diagnosis in a young woman with a positive pregnancy test, 6 weeks amenorrhoea, lower abdominal pain and vaginal bleeding essentially lies between miscarriage and ectopic pregnancy. Traditionally, spontaneous miscarriage is divided into three clinical categories (Fig. 30.1). The first is threatened miscarriage, where there is painless vaginal bleeding which may settle spontaneously with a continuing pregnancy or progress to an inevitable miscarriage. The second is an inevitable miscarriage, where there is bleeding and pain associated with cervical dilatation, which will progress to the third type, (in)complete miscarriage, where part or all of the products of conception have been passed vaginally. Ultrasound examination, however, will produce an alternative classification for spontaneous miscarriage, including blighted ovum, missed miscarriage and live miscarriage. Blighted ovum is an anembryonic pregnancy where only a gestation sac and placental tissue can be identified but no fetus ever forms.

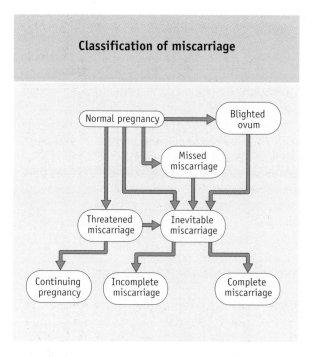

Classification of miscarriage

Fig. 30.1   Classification of miscarriage.

A missed miscarriage is a situation where the fetus can be seen on ultrasound but there is an absent fetal heart pulsation indicating that the fetus has perished prior to miscarriage per se occurring. Live miscarriage is a situation where the fetal heart pulsation may be identified shortly before expulsion of the products of conception, implying that the fetal loss is a consequence rather than a direct cause of the process.

Ectopic pregnancy also presents with lower abdominal pain and vaginal bleeding after an episode of amenorrhoea with a positive pregnancy test. The commonest site is the fallopian tube, in which >95% are sited. The villus trophoblast rapidly invades the mucosa of the fallopian tube and, as the pregnancy grows, bleeding and tubal rupture can occur.

What features would you look for on examination?

The key differential diagnosis for the above patient is therefore that of inevitable or (in)complete miscarriage or ectopic pregnancy. The diagnosis of spontaneous miscarriage is usually straightforward. Clinical examination and pelvic examination should assess for abdominal and adnexal tenderness, the presence of cervical dilatation and uterine size. In inevitable and incomplete miscarriage the cervix may be found to be open and sometimes products of conception can be found passing through the cervix or in the vagina.

In ectopic pregnancy there may be more abdominal tenderness associated with peritoneal irritation, manifesting as rebound tenderness. The uterus may be of normal size. It should be noted that a patient in this situation will be at high risk of major haemorrhage and possible hypovolaemic shock.

What investigations, if any, are required?

Ultrasound scan of the pelvis (Fig. 30.2) and confirmation of pregnancy, ideally by measuring beta-hCG, should be carried out. Ectopic pregnancy is principally diagnosed by biochemical confirmation of pregnancy and the finding of an

(a)
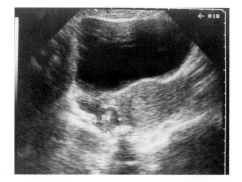

(b)
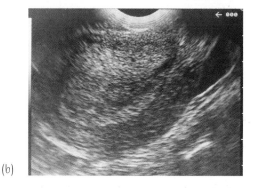

Fig. 30.2 *Ultrasound scan showing ectopic pregnancy. (a) Transabdominal scan showing empty uterus with a complex mass in the right adnexa measuring 21 × 22 mm. (b) Transvaginal scan showing absence of gestational sac in the uterus and decidual reaction with marked endometrial thickening. There is free fluid in the pouch of Douglas (blood will be found there in ruptured ectopic pregnancy).*

empty uterus on ultrasound scan, and not by the direct identification of the ectopic, although this may sometimes be found. Ultrasound can detect an intrauterine pregnancy, and the presence of an intrauterine pregnancy virtually excludes ectopic pregnancy because heterotopic pregnancy, i.e. a combined intra- and extrauterine pregnancy, is exceedingly rare in normal conceptions. Thus, a beta-hCG level above the discriminatory level for an intrauterine pregnancy to be identified on ultrasound, coupled with an empty uterus on ultrasound scan, implies that an ectopic pregnancy is present. Transvaginal ultrasound provides a better image, and the potential for the earlier detection of ectopic pregnancy, than transabdominal ultrasound. Laparocopy will confirm the diagnosis of ectopic pregnancy.

On examination you find no abnormality on abdominal palpation and, in particular, no tenderness. On vaginal examination, however, you find blood clot in the vagina and products of conception are present in the cervix, which is dilated. What is the diagnosis and how would you manage the situation?

With the presence of products of conception in the cervical os, it would appear that this patient has had an inevitable miscarriage, which is in the process of progressing to a complete or incomplete miscarriage. Products present in the cervix should be removed digitally, as these can sometimes provoke an extreme vagal reaction. Thereafter the patient will usually require surgical evacuation of the uterus and arrangements should be made to take her to theatre for this to be carried out. Should major haemorrhage occur in the course of such a miscarriage, it would be usual to treat the patient with intravenous fluids and blood if necessary. Ergometrine in a dose of 0.25–0.5 mg can be given intravenously if bleeding is continuing. When evacuation is undertaken it is best performed digitally to avoid the risk of perforation, although a gentle curettage may be required to ensure that the uterus is empty. Intravenous oxytocin or ergometrine may be given intraoperatively to prevent or control bleeding. If there is any suspicion of the miscarriage being complicated by sepsis, appropriate antibiotic therapy will be required. If serious sepsis exists, evacuation should be delayed until the sepsis has been controlled, usually after 24 h or so of antibiotic therapy, to avoid the risk of disseminating the infection and provoking septicaemia.

Anaemia

A para 3+0 at 32 weeks gestation complains of excessive tiredness at the antenatal clinic. She has no other symptoms and the pregnancy is uncomplicated. Full blood count is performed and the haemoglobin is found to be 9.5 g%.

What is the most likely diagnosis?

The most likely diagnosis is iron deficiency anaemia, as over 90% of anaemia in pregnancy is due to iron deficiency associated with depleted iron stores. Folate deficiency may coexist along with iron deficiency, as both can be associated with poor diet. When both folate and iron are deficient the effects of folate deficiency are usually obscured by the iron deficiency. True vitamin B_{12} deficiency is extremely rare in pregnancy.

It is noteworthy that the physiological changes of pregnancy result in an apparent 'physiological anaemia'. This is due to a substantial increase in plasma volume of around 50%, with a concomitant increase in red cell mass, which is usually of the order of 25%. Thus, as plasma volume increases by a greater proportion than the red cell mass, the haemoglobin concentration will fall as a result of dilution. This effect is maximal at 32 weeks gestation. It is generally accepted that haemoglobin should not fall below 10.5–11 g/dl at any time during normal pregnancy.

What further information is required to make the diagnosis?

Further information that would be required to determine the type of anaemia from which this patient is suffering would be the parameters available on full blood count: mean corpuscular haemoglobin (MCH), mean corpuscular volume (MCV) and mean corpuscular haemoglobin concentration (MCHC). All of these parameters would be reduced in iron deficiency anaemia. (A differential diagnosis of thalassaemia should also be considered. This will show markedly reduced MCV and MCH but a normal or only slightly reduced MCHC). A blood film should also be requested, which will show a hypochromic microcytic picture in well-established iron deficiency anaemia. However, characteristic red cell morphology in iron deficiency anaemia is a relatively late development and will be preceded by a reduction in the MCV and subsequently a reduction in the MCHC. Women entering pregnancy with grossly depleted iron stores, perhaps from previous pregnancies following which iron stores have not been allowed to recover, may rapidly develop anaemia with clear evidence of iron deficiency on the red cell indices. Where there is suspicion of iron deficiency anaemia and the red cell indices are not diagnostic, serum ferritin and total iron binding capacity are useful measures of iron status. A concentration of serum ferritin of < 12 mg/l is compatible with iron deficiency. It is noteworthy that serum ferritin falls over the course of a pregnancy and this must be taken into account in the interpretation of such data. Serum iron and percentage saturation of the total iron binding capacity may be useful. These measurements may fluctuate widely; they are affected by iron ingestion and thus are less helpful in diagnosis than serum ferritin. However, a reduced total iron binding capacity saturation and reduced serum iron are compatible with iron deficiency anaemia in pregnancy.

The mean corpuscular volume is 71 fl (normal range: 75–99 fl), the MCH is 24 pg (normal range: 27–31 pg) and the

MCHC 28 g/dl (normal range: 32–36 g/dl). Does this confirm your diagnosis and what treatment would you prescribe?

These indices are compatible with iron deficiency anaemia: appropriate treatment would be oral iron supplementation, which would usually be prescribed along with folic acid supplements. It may also be useful to prescribe vitamin C together with the iron as this may enhance absorption; alternatively, the iron could be taken with a drink of fresh orange juice. Where poor compliance or intolerance of oral iron preparations occurs, parenteral iron may be required; however, this is uncommon. Clearly at 32 weeks gestation there is an urgent need to increase the haemoglobin concentration in anticipation of the haemostatic challenge of delivery. Thus, the patient should be followed up and it would be anticipated that, with appropriate correction of the iron deficiency, haemoglobin should rise by between 0.8 and 1 g/dl/week. A commonly prescribed regimen is 200 mg ferrous sulphate 2–3 times a day taken with 50 mg vitamin C. In addition, 5 mg folic acid should be administered daily.

Epilepsy

A 21 year old primigravida attends for booking at 9 weeks gestation by menstrual dates and ultrasound. She suffers from epilepsy, which takes the form of grand mal seizures. She takes carbamazepine to prevent convulsions and normally only has one to two seizures per year while on treatment, although she had a convulsion 1 week prior to her attending the clinic. She has suffered from epilepsy since the age of 7 years. She has read that carbamazepine may be associated with fetal abnormalities and she is very anxious about this.

She seeks your advice, specifically as to whether she should stop carbamazepine now, and also wishes to know what the implications of her condition and its drug therapy are for the pregnancy and its management.

With regard to her specific query about stopping the carbamazepine, what must be weighed up is the risk of fetal abnormality from the carbamazepine versus the risk of seizures. All commonly used anticonvulsants are associated with fetal abnormalities (Fig. 32.1), and although carbamazepine appears to be associated with less risk of neural tube defect than sodium valproate, there is

Fetal abnormality	
Major	Neural tube defect
	Cardiac defect
	Cleft lip and palate
Minor	Club foot
	Hypospadias
Dysmorphic feature	Hypertelorism
	Long philtrum
	Low-set ears
	Wide mouth
	Irregular teeth
	Hypoplasia of distal phalanges and nails

Fig. 32.1   *Fetal abnormalities associated with antiepileptic drugs.*

nonetheless a significant risk of fetal abnormality when this drug is used in the first trimester. Monotherapy with anticonvulsants is associated with around a 7% risk of fetal abnormality. Information on newer anticonvulsant agents is limited. Lamotrigine appears to be safer on initial reports but data are too limited to provide any conclusive evidence. Topiramate and gabapentin are teratogenic in animal studies. The main abnormality of concern is a neural tube defect, such as spina bifida. The neural tube, however, closes at 7 weeks gestation and therefore stopping carbamazepine at 9 weeks gestation would not prevent a neural tube defect. Thus, with regard to the major fetal abnormality that the patient need be concerned about, there would be no benefit from stopping the carbamazepine at 9 weeks gestation. If she were to have uncontrolled grand mal seizures, this might provoke fetal hypoxia, which itself could be hazardous. In addition, a significant number of women with epilepsy die in pregnancy and poorly controlled seizures are a risk factor. The UK Confidential Enquiry into Maternal Deaths reports these deaths and a recurrent feature is women with epilepsy dying in the bath from drowning, presumably following a seizure. Some deaths in pregnancy are likely to be classified as sudden unexplained death in epilepsy (SUDEP). Thus, weighing up these risks, it is clear that your advice should be to continue the carbamazepine, and the risks and benefits should be discussed with her.

It is noteworthy that she had a seizure a week prior to being seen. This may reflect a lack of compliance on her part because of her anxiety about fetal abnormality. This emphasizes the need to communicate accurately to the patient the balance of risk, specifically indicating that any risk of serious fetal abnormality has now passed and the main risk would come from uncontrolled seizures. It also highlights the benefit of prepregnancy care, where these issues can be addressed before conception.

Ideally such patients should conceive while on folic acid supplements. Folic acid supplements have been shown to reduce the risk of neural tube defects. This has not been proven in conjunction with anticonvulsant therapy. However, it is prudent to prescribe folic acid supplements for patients on anticonvulsants associated with neural tube defects, especially as many women with epilepsy have low folic acid levels due to anticonvulsant drugs increasing hepatic metabolism. It is usual to prescribe 5 mg of folic acid daily. Clearly such information and advice is best imparted prepregnancy and the ideal situation is for a patient with epilepsy on anticonvulsant drugs to be seen for prepregnancy counselling. If prepregnancy counselling were to occur, it would also be useful to review the drug therapy in terms of whether or not it is needed; also, if the patient is not on monotherapy, consider reducing to one drug as multiple drug therapy enhances the risks, such that if the patient is on three anticonvulsants the risk of fetal abnormality is of the order of 25%. This clearly does not apply in the present case.

With regard to the risks and management of the rest of her pregnancy, we should first consider that of fetal abnormality. Clearly no preventive measures can be taken at 9 weeks gestation regarding neural tube defects, and the focus has to be on diagnosis. She should be offered alpha-fetoprotein screening for neural tube defects, and a detailed ultrasound scan at 18 weeks gestation to assess the fetus for any anatomical abnormality such as spina bifida or cleft palate.

Drug therapy with enzyme-inducing anticonvulsant agents, such as carbemazepine, can also cause relative deficiency of vitamin K in the neonate; this can be prevented by vitamin K supplements from 36 weeks gestation in a dose of 20 mg once a day to the mother. As vitamin K is a water-soluble vitamin it is easily and readily absorbed from oral administration. Following delivery, the baby should also receive vitamin K supplements. These measures should minimize the risk of haemorrhagic disease of the newborn, which is a risk for patients on anticonvulsant therapy. Enzyme-inducing agents also enhance steroid metabolism. This has implications for prescription of steroids; for example, double the dose of dexamethasone or betamethasone normally used to enhance fetal lung maturity is required in women on enzyme-inducing anticonvulsant agents. If the combined oral contraceptive pill is used after delivery, a pill containing 50 µg of ethinyloestradiol should be used and the pill-free interval reduced to 4 days (Fig. 32.2).

**Hormonal contraception for women taking
enzyme-inducing anticonvulsants**

Combined oral contraceptive pill: 50µg ethinyl oestradiol pill should be used.

May require even higher dose of oestradiol if breakthrough bleeding occurs.

Reduce pill-free interval to 4 days and use four packs of combined oral contraceptive pills consecutively to enhance contraceptive cover. This may also prevent seizures if they are hormonally triggered at the time of menstruation.

Progesterone-only pill: should only be used if there is no other acceptable method, and doubling of the daily dose may be effective.

Depo-progestogen: reduce dosing interval from 12 weeks to 10 weeks for Depo-Provera®.

Fig. 32.2   *Hormonal contraception for women taking enzyme-inducing anticonvulsants.*

Pregnancy does not influence seizure frequency in patients with epilepsy in any predictable way. Some studies have found no change in the seizure frequency, others an increase and yet others a decrease. There is also no pattern from pregnancy to pregnancy. Given the various factors that can influence seizure frequency in pregnancy, such as hormonal changes, altered drug distribution volume and excretion, issues of compliance, vomiting and so on, this is not surprising. Seizures may be provoked by stressful situations and sleep deprivation, both of which can occur in pregnancy and particularly at the time of labour, when 1–2% of women with epilepsy will have a seizure. Thus, the patient may face stresses that could precipitate convulsions.

Pregnancy also alters total plasma levels of the anticonvulsant drugs. There is an increased volume of distribution, a marked alteration in plasma protein binding and increased clearance. In the case of carbamazepine, this results in a substantial decrease in total drug level and a more modest reduction in free drug levels, thus total drug levels are a poor guide to the actual levels of the free drug in pregnancy. As it is the levels of the free drug that are important, this must be taken into account when monitoring plasma levels. An important benefit of monitoring plasma

levels of anticonvulsants in pregnancy is to ensure compliance. As noted above, many patients reduce their compliance, often in an attempt to prevent any harm coming to the fetus from the drugs. Should the patient have a convulsion and her therapy be adjusted by way of an increased dose, then in the situation where the patient has not previously been taking the drugs through non-compliance and this is unknown to the doctor caring for her, potential toxic problems can ensue. In addition, as pregnancy alters the handling of anticonvulsants, it may be appropriate to adjust the dose should gross alterations in drug levels occur, in order to prevent convulsions due to subtherapeutic drug levels. There is also an argument, however, that in the absence of toxicity the dose should be adjusted to maintain the patient seizure-free rather than using a biochemical assessment. In this patient's case it may be worth monitoring the drug levels because there may be reservations about compliance as she has had a recent seizure and we are uncertain as to whether seizure frequency will increase or not. Information on plasma drug levels may be advantageous in this situation. Postpartum it is important to take account of any increase in dose during the pregnancy, as dosage should be adjusted to the prepregnancy dose.

Breast feeding is not contraindicated but specific measures need to be taken to avoid harm to the baby during feeding should a convulsion occur. Such measures include breast feeding while sitting on the floor with cushions around her and having the partner or another person present. She should avoid bathing the baby or preparing bottles when she is alone in case a seizure occurs.

Compared with the infant of a woman without epilepsy, the infant will have an increased risk, around fourfold, of developing epilepsy.

Systemic lupus erythematosus

Your colleague in the Rheumatology Department refers a patient with systemic lupus erythematosus (SLE) to you for prepregnancy advice. She is 28 years of age and has had SLE for 7 years. It has manifested itself with arthritis and the Raynaud phenomenon. At initial presentation the patient had renal involvement, but at the present time renal function is satisfactory and there is no proteinuria. The disease is currently quiescent and she is on 10 mg prednisolone/day. She uses a non-steroidal anti-inflammatory agent when her arthritis is troublesome.

What are the points you would discuss at prepregnancy counselling?

SLE is an autoimmune connective tissue disease with autoantibodies that can cause specific cytotoxic damage, such as haemolytic anaemia or thrombocytopenia, and immune complex problems leading to inflammatory lesions that can affect the kidneys, the skin and the central nervous system. Perhaps the major immune complex implicated in this mechanism is DNA–anti-DNA, which can produce arthritis as described in this patient. Arthritis is a common manifestation and it is generally non-deforming, in contrast to the arthritis found in rheumatoid arthritis. Clinical evidence of glomerulonephritis can be found in over half of cases of SLE. A variety of glomerular lesions can be seen in this condition and the prognosis appears to be better with mesangial and membranous glomerular nephritis and poor in proliferative glomerular nephritis. Antinuclear factor is found in over 95% of patients with SLE but anti-DNA antibodies are more specific and can be used to monitor disease activity along with the complement components C3 and C4. In particular, depressed complement and high levels of anti-native DNA, indicating disease activity, can be associated with lupus nephritis.

Perhaps the first thing to consider is the effect of SLE on fertility; there is no evidence of significantly impaired fertility rates in women with SLE.

SLE is associated with an increased risk of fetal loss due to a high rate of spontaneous miscarriage, intrauterine death and premature delivery because of pregnancy complications. IUGR is also more common and there is an increased risk of pre-eclampsia. Patients with a background history of lupus nephritis may be at particular risk, as are those who enter pregnancy with active disease. It would therefore be useful to check her renal function and establish if she has hypertension. The increased fetal loss and placental problems may be due to decidual vasculitis compromising placental blood supply, or to an abnormal immune response to the invading trophoblast.

A particular problem is the presence of lupus anticoagulant and/or anticardiolipin antibodies, which are associated with a higher incidence of vascular problems and adverse pregnancy outcomes, including maternal venous and arterial thrombosis, recurrent miscarriage, placental infarction, IUGR and pre-eclampsia. It is therefore important to establish whether or not she has anticardiolipin antibodies or lupus anticoagulant; if results of investigations are not available, these should be checked at the time of prepregnancy counselling. In addition, if negative they should be repeated during the pregnancy as sometimes these antibodies are only found during pregnancy. Between 5 and 18% of women with SLE will have anticardiolipin antibodies or lupus anticoagulant. Lupus anticoagulant is an antibody to phospholipids that interferes with the activation of prothrombin by the prothrombin converting complex of factor Va, factor Xa, calcium and lipid. A variety of laboratory tests exist to assess its presence, such as the activated partial thromboplastin time, the dilute prothrombin time or the Russell's viper venom time. Although this condition is associated with prolongation of laboratory tests of coagulation in vitro, in vivo it is associated with thrombotic problems, which can occur at the level of the placental bed, causing the problems discussed above. Anticardiolipin antibodies are antibodies specifically directed against phospholipids and, while often existing with lupus anticoagulant, these antibodies are not one and the same. High levels of anticardiolipin antibody are powerful predictors of fetal compromise and high risk of fetal death in women with SLE. Low-dose aspirin may be of benefit in patients with lupus anticoagulant and anticardiolipin antibodies to prevent some of the complications. Prophylactic doses of low molecular weight heparin combined with low-dose aspirin are of value for recurrent fetal loss associated with lupus anticoagulant and/or anticardiolipin antibodies. Clearly heparin should be used if there is a past history of deep venous thrombosis.

It is also important to screen for the presence of the anti-Ro and anti-La antibodies as these are important risk factors for neonatal lupus syndrome. This is a passively acquired autoimmune condition characterized by lupus dermatitis and a variety of systemic and haematological abnormalities. This syndrome will occur in about 5% of babies where the mother has anti-Ro. In particular, anti-Ro can attack the conducting system of the fetal heart and can lead to congenital heart block, which in turn may lead to intrauterine death. Congenital heart block occurs in about 4% of pregnancies where the mother has anti-Ro antibodies. If serology for these antibodies is not available from previous investigation, this should be checked at the time of prepregnancy counselling.

Once the information on anticardiolipin antibodies, anti-Ro and anti-La and renal function are available, her risk of complications can be more accurately assessed. These risks must be clearly communicated to her to allow her and her partner to make an informed choice as to whether or not to proceed with attempting to conceive. The background of renal involvement will put this woman at particular risk of complications in the pregnancy.

She should be advised that it is optimal for her to conceive when the disease is quiescent, and it would appear from the history that such a state exists at the time of referral. Drug therapy should be employed at the minimal dose to maintain disease control. Steroids can safely be used in pregnancy. There is no evidence of teratogenicity in the human. Although their administration in high doses may cause adrenal suppression in the neonate, this is very unusual in practice and when it occurs it is of a transient nature and can be easily treated with steroid supplements. There is an increased risk of steroid-related side-effects for the mother, such as weight gain, gestational diabetes and osteoporosis. The overriding interest in this situation is quiescent disease in the mother: steroids should not be withheld. Thus, she should be reassured with regard to her steroid therapy in pregnancy. Non-steroidal anti-inflammatory drugs should be avoided if possible. Although they are not teratogenic they are associated with oligohydramnios owing to their effects on the fetal kidney and there is a risk of premature closure of the ductus arteriosus. They may also put the fetus and neonate at risk of haemorrhage, as they inhibit platelet function. If they have to be used because of arthritis, the course should be as short as possible and liquor volume should be monitored. Ideally, they should not be used after 32 weeks gestation.

To minimise the risks of SLE, it would appear prudent to treat her with low-dose aspirin in a dose of 75 mg once a day at least from the end of the first trimester, even if she does not have anticardiolipin antibodies and lupus anticoagulant. If anticardiolipin antibodies or lupus anticoagulant is found, then consideration should be given to thromboprophylaxis. This should certainly be given postpartum, when the risk may be highest. It is debatable whether, in the absence of a previous thrombosis, antenatal prophylaxis is required; however, this should be considered for each individual case. If considered necessary, low molecular weight heparin is usually employed.

The effects of pregnancy on SLE should also be discussed. Exacerbations and flare-ups brought on by pregnancy have been reported, particularly in the first and second trimesters; however, whether pregnancy actually increases the risk of flare remains controversial. There is recent evidence to suggest that, if pregnancy begins in a patient with inactive disease, there is a reduced chance of flare associated with the pregnancy.

Management of the pregnancy should be outlined. This will involve careful monitoring of the pregnancy, starting with an accurate determination of gestational age and the introduction of low-dose aspirin by around 12 weeks gestation, or at diagnosis of pregnancy if anticardiolipin antibodies are present. In the second trimester uterine artery blood flow should be assessed by Doppler ultrasound: a persistent notching pattern may identify fetuses at increased risk of adverse perinatal outcome. Fetal growth should be monitored from around 24–26 weeks gestation by ultrasound, and umbilical artery blood flow assessed using Doppler ultrasound. Regular assessment of fetal well-being

should also be made from late in the second trimester, using either biophysical profiles or cardiotocographs in conjunction with liquor volume if there is any disturbance of fetal growth or pregnancy complications. The intensity of monitoring for fetal well-being will depend on the nature and severity of any complications, such as growth restriction.

The patient must be watched carefully for development of superimposed pre-eclampsia and worsening of her lupus. It can often be difficult to determine whether the onset of problems such as oedema and hypertension are due to superimposed pre-eclampsia or a flare-up of lupus nephritis. The occurrence of these features, in the absence of other clinical evidence of a flare in SLE and increased levels of DNA antibodies and reduced complement levels, suggests superimposed pre-eclampsia. Conversely, elevated DNA antibodies, suppressed complement levels and granular casts in the urine would favour the diagnosis of a flare-up in the SLE.

The timing and mode of delivery will depend very much on the development of any complications in the pregnancy, but in the absence of complications vaginal delivery is not contraindicated. She will need parenteral steroid supplements to cover the stress of labour and delivery. Clearly, these women have a significantly higher risk of caesarean section because of problems such as pre-eclampsia and IUGR.

Following discussion with you, she decides that she does not want to proceed with a pregnancy at the present time but seeks your advice with regard to contraception. She has been using barrier methods up to this time but feels, in view of the implications of a pregnancy, that she would like a more secure form of contraception. She asks specifically if she can go on the oral contraceptive pill. What is your advice?

The oral contraceptive is generally not used in patients with SLE, as the oestrogen component can provoke worsening of symptoms or a flare-up of the SLE. There is also evidence of increased incidence of thrombosis, vasculitis and high blood pressure in women using combined oral contraceptives; thus, she should be discouraged from using the combined oral contraceptive pill. The progesterone-only pill may be an option for her, or she could continue with barrier methods. The IUCD may be of value but there is a small risk of recurrent infections, particularly if she is on steroid therapy.

Pregnancy in the haemophilia carrier

A 26 year old primigravida is referred to your antenatal clinic at 10 weeks gestation by menstrual dates and ultrasound scan. She tells you that her father suffers from haemophilia A, for which he had a joint replacement because of haemophiliac arthropathy. In addition, she believes that her father suffers from some form of hepatitis that she thinks was related to blood product administration.

Is she likely to have a bleeding problem?

The genes for haemophilia A and B are carried on the X chromosome; thus, daughters of haemophiliac fathers are obligate carriers of this genetic defect. In contrast, if the mother is a carrier, then half her daughters will be carriers. Thus, this patient is an obligate carrier for haemophilia A, i.e. deficiency of factor VIII. Such carriers will generally have a normal gene in the other X chromosome and, because of this, they will usually have coagulation factor activity within the normal range (> 50 iu/dl). This is sufficient for normal haemostasis, so the majority of carriers do not have significant bleeding problems. Nonetheless, bleeding problems can develop in the small number of carriers who have coagulation factor activities of < 40 iu/dl. Such carriers may have low coagulation factor activities due to extreme lyonization of the factor VIII gene or coinheritance of a variant of von Willebrand factor allele.

The risk of bleeding problems in haemophilia carriers relates to low levels of factor VIII. In normal pregnancy, the haemostatic system changes in favour of coagulation. There are substantial increases in fibrinogen, factor VIII and von Willebrand factor occurring progressively through pregnancy. Haemophilia carriers also exhibit this increase in factor VIII and von Willebrand factor during pregnancy. Thus, even if they enter pregnancy with abnormally low levels of factor VIII, in the majority of cases the increase in factor VIII will usually be sufficient to avoid any risk of excessive bleeding due to their carrier status. Where such an increase in factor VIII fails to occur, the haemophilia carrier will be at increased risk of bleeding in the course of normal or operative delivery and may therefore require treatment to prevent this. In this case it is important to establish the factor VIII level in order to answer her question accurately.

What issues would you raise with her and why would prepregnancy counselling have been of value in this patient?

Ideally, it is important to see haemophilia carriers before they embark on pregnancy. Features that should be discussed include the possibility of pre-natal diagnosis (if the fetus is female she has a 50/50 chance of being a carrier, and, if male, a 50/50 chance of being affected with haemophilia). She should also be advised as to the possible complications in the pregnancy should she be at risk of bleeding; thus, it would be important to identify the plasma concentration of factor VIII prepregnancy and also to indicate that this should be monitored during pregnancy. If the baseline level is within the normal range, she can be reassured that she is unlikely to have any haemostatic problems relating to her carrier status during her pregnancy. However, if the factor VIII level is low, this would require careful monitoring through pregnancy. In the unlikely event that it failed to rise into the normal range, then treatment might be necessary. Often blood product therapy can be avoided by use of a desmopressin (DDAVP®) infusion, which can stimulate an increase in factor VIII levels in advance of delivery. If she is at risk of requiring blood product therapy, for example if she does not respond to DDAVP, then good practice is to provide immunization of such women against hepatitis A and B because of risk of viral transmission. Good liaison should also be established with the regional haemophilia unit, and ideally this should start prepregnancy. Invasive procedures such as chorionic villus sampling and amniocentesis may place her at risk of haemorrhagic problems. This must be weighed against the potential benefits of such investigations but risk of bleeding can be minimized by treatment such as DDAVP infusion.

Carriers with low activities of factor VIII may also be at particular risk of obstetric bleeding problems in the first or second trimester (before factor VIII levels normalize) should miscarriage occur. Sexing of the fetus by ultrasound examination at around 18 weeks gestation is of value.

You explain the issues of prenatal diagnosis and management of pregnancy and she indicates that she does not wish formal prenatal diagnosis, as she would not want to terminate the pregnancy even if she were carrying an affected male fetus. However, she does request a detailed scan to assess the fetal sex in the second trimester, as she says she would feel reassured should the fetus be female. You organize this and, in addition to routine booking bloods, you check her factor VIII level and take a detailed history to determine whether or not she has had any haemostatic problems. She denies any such problems but does mention that she remembers her mother telling her that she had a problem with bleeding after she had a tonsillectomy as a child. On further detailed questioning, she feels she may bruise easily. She has not previously had any formal assessment of her plasma factor VIII concentration. You warn her that, should she have any complications, and in particular any bleeding complications, she is to get in touch with the hospital quickly. You arrange to see her around the time of her next ultrasound scan. At that visit the ultrasound scan shows that the fetus appears to be a female and your patient is reassured. However, the regional haemophilia centre have returned the investigations of her coagulation status to you and these indicate that her factor VIII level at the time of her booking visit was 19 iu/dl. The consultant at the haemophilia unit has also written to you to indicate that this will require careful monitoring through the pregnancy, and that, should it not increase, treatment may be required in the course of delivery. You communicate this to the patient and also arrange another appointment for her to see the consultant at the regional haemophilia unit.

At her next visit to the antenatal clinic, some 6 weeks later, she is anxious with regard to delivery. What are the important issues with regard to delivery in haemophilia carriers?

The usual goal in carriers of haemophilia A and B is to have an uncomplicated vaginal delivery. It is usual to ensure that an experienced obstetrician is involved both in managing the delivery and their postpartum care. The fetus is at risk of being affected by, or being a carrier of, haemophilia; thus the use of fetal scalp electrodes, fetal scalp blood sampling and any potentially traumatic forceps delivery should be avoided. The ventouse must not be used in any situation where the fetus is at risk of bleeding. Should the labour become complicated, early recourse to caesarean section is preferable for the fetus, to avoid any bleeding problems. There is a risk of traumatic vaginal delivery being associated with haemorrhage within the brain and subsequent handicap.

In addition, it is important to discuss delivery with the anaesthetist, as epidural anaesthesia in haemophilia carriers with low factor VIII levels is a controversial issue and many anaesthetists would be reluctant to use it. Furthermore, parenteral analgesia must be administered subcutaneously or intravenously as intramuscular injections in a patient with a relatively low factor VIII concentration may cause significant haematoma. It would also appear prudent to avoid non-steroidal anti-inflammatory drugs, which can inhibit platelet function, in the postpartum management of carriers with significantly reduced factor VIII coagulant activities, as the combination of a defect in platelet function and a defect in the intrinsic co-agulation system might place the patient at an increased risk of bleeding.

At delivery, a cord blood sample should be taken to help to determine whether a male fetus is affected; however, as some haemostatic factors are present at relatively reduced concentrations in neonates, it may be difficult to diagnose accurately a mild-to-moderate inherited bleeding defect at birth and repeat examination may be necessary. Thus, intramuscular injections should be avoided in male fetuses of haemophilia carriers unless it is clear that the baby is unaffected. Prophylactic vitamin K should be administered orally to these neonates (treating the mother with oral vitamin K, 20 mg/day, in the weeks leading up to delivery may also help) and immunizations should be given subcutaneously or intradermally, avoiding the intramuscular route. Both the mother and child should be followed up by the local haemophilia unit.

At 36 weeks gestation, factor VIIIC activity has risen to 55 iu/dl but the fetus has a breech presentation. You discuss the options with regard to delivery and external cephalic version; however, she prefers delivery by elective caesarean section. This is performed uneventfully under general anaesthesia and a healthy female fetus weighing 3.1 kg is delivered. Two weeks later the mother returns with bleeding per vaginam over the preceding 12 h. Prior to this she was complaining of offensive discharge and some lower abdominal pain. What is the likely diagnosis and how would you manage it?

Bleeding 2 weeks after caesarean section with a history of offensive lochia suggestive of infection is likely to indicate postpartum endometritis. Retained products of conception is unlikely given that she had a caesarean section. Management should include ultrasound scan to confirm that the uterus is empty, high vaginal and endocervical swabs for bacteriological analysis, and prescription of broad-spectrum antibiotics while awaiting bacteriological culture and sensitivity. In this particular patient, assessment of her coagulation status will also be required because the factor VIII concentration is likely to have declined below the pregnancy value and could also contribute to the bleeding and require specific haemostatic treatment with blood products or DDAVP.

Hyperthyroidism

A 32 year old patient with a history of hyperthyroidism characterized as Graves disease attends for prepregnancy advice. She is worried that her hyperthyroidism, or the drugs used to treat it, may have an effect on the pregnancy. She is controlled on carbimazole at the time of the consultation.

What effect does pregnancy have on thyroid function and how does this influence the interpretation of her thyroid function tests?

The physiological changes in pregnancy can mimic thyroid symptoms. Pregnancy itself causes alterations in the structure and function of the thyroid gland that can produce diagnostic confusion in the interpretation of thyroid function tests; however, the overall control of the thyroid gland is unaltered in normal pregnancy. The change in the thyroid function tests is due predominantly to increased binding of the active thyroid hormones, T_3 and T_4, by thyroid binding globulin, which increases dramatically in concentration in the first trimester. This alteration in thyroid binding globulin is oestrogen dependent. Thus, total T_3 and total T_4 are substantially increased in pregnancy; however, free T_3 and T_4 measurements usually stay within the normal range. Similarly, TSH usually stays within the normal range. In interpreting thyroid function tests in pregnancy it is therefore important to measure free T_4 and TSH.

Outline the risks of pregnancy to this patient and indicate how she should be managed.

Hyperthyroidism is a relatively common medical disorder and may occur in 1 in 500 pregnancies. The vast majority of cases are diagnosed and treated prior to pregnancy (indeed uncontrolled disease can lead to ovulation failure and infertility). Most cases of hyperthyroidism are secondary to Graves disease, an autoimmune disorder with circulating thyroid stimulating antibodies being present. Occasionally some improvement can occur in pregnancy; however, the situation may worsen postpartum.

As noted above, some of the signs and symptoms of hyperthyroidism, such as tachycardia, heat intolerance and ejection systolic murmurs, are similar to those seen with the normal hyperdynamic cardiovascular state of pregnancy. Thus, it is important not to rely on clinical features alone and thyroid function tests should be regularly assessed. The frequency of testing will depend on the individual case but should be at least every 3 months.

Untreated or inadequately treated hyperthyroidism in pregnancy is associated with an increased risk of miscarriage, IUGR and preterm labour. With regard to the mother, the main concern is uncontrolled disease, which may, in its more severe form, present as a 'thyroid storm' — a major medical problem. Thyroid storms can be precipitated by infection or stress and are characterized by hyperpyrexia and tachycardia. Atrial fibrillation may occur. Cardiovascular problems can lead to high-output cardiac failure. Gastro-intestinal upset with vomiting and diarrhoea and central nervous system dysfunction can also occur. This situation is extremely rare. In patients who are well controlled with antithyroid drugs the maternal and fetal outcome is not usually influenced by the disease.

The usual drugs used to control hyperthyroidism in the United Kingdom are carbimazole, propylthiouracil and propranolol. Carbimazole and propylthiouracil inhibit thyroid hormone synthesis, while propanolol decreases the adrenergic symptoms. It is important to indicate to the mother prepregnancy the need for continued therapy during pregnancy and the need for regular assessment by thyroid function studies. Thus, she should continue on her carbimazole or propylthiouracil therapy through pregnancy, being maintained on the lowest dose of drug that keeps her clinically and biochemically euthyroid. Once the thyrotoxicosis is under control there is no need for propranolol therapy and this is not usually required in pregnancy except in newly diagnosed cases.

With regard to the fetus, all the drugs used to control hyperthyroidism cross the placenta and may therefore affect fetal thyroid function. Less propylthiouracil than carbimazole crosses the placenta; however, both agents are satisfactory and there is no need to switch from carbimazole to propylthiouracil. In high doses both agents can inhibit fetal thyroid function and induce a fetal goitre, but at maintainence doses of ≤15 mg of carbimazole a day or 150 mg propylthiouracil a day no fetal problems are likely to be encountered.

These drugs are not associated with teratogenesis, although carbimazole has been associated with aplasia cutis, a condition where small defects in the skin occur. These are usually on the head and produce a coin-shaped defect in the scalp. This, however, is rare. Maintenance doses of antithyroid drugs are safe for breast feeding

Perhaps the main consideration is the transfer of thyroid stimulating antibodies from the mother to the fetus, which can provoke hyperthyroidism in the fetus. This is manifest as fetal tachycardia, goitre and IUGR, but maternal antithyroid medication will usually prevent severe problems in utero. Neonatal thyrotoxicosis occurs in around 10% of the babies of mothers with Graves disease. It is usually transient, lasting only weeks to at most 2–3 months following delivery. The maternal administration of carbimazole may mask such a problem at birth and it may not be apparent for several days.

Radioactive iodine should not be used in pregnancy as the fetal thyroid will concentrate it, which may have serious consequences for the fetus. Partial thyroidectomy may be required in pregnancies in which patients do not respond to medication, in those who develop an intolerance to drug therapy or those who have a symptomatic goitre with dysphagia. Before surgery patients are usually prepared with 7–10 days iodine therapy to decrease the vascularity of the thyroid gland and prevent thyroid storm.

It is usual in pregnancy to monitor fetal growth by ultrasound, with monitoring being increased to regular fetal well-being assessments if there is a suspicion of any disturbance in fetal growth. The fetal heart rate should be noted and the neck scanned for the development of goitre.

There are no special requirements for labour in these patients with controlled thyrotoxicosis in the absence of major complications and they should be considered 'normal' for the purposes of intrapartum care. In the postpartum period the patient and those caring for her should be aware of the possibility of worsening disease following delivery. There may also be a need to adjust the medication dose if this has been increased during pregnancy.

Diabetes

A 30 year old school teacher attends you at 6 weeks gestation for a booking visit. She is an insulin-dependent diabetic and has already visited you for prepregnancy advice and also has seen the diabetic physician. She has been trying to conceive for several months and had endeavoured to maintain good glycaemic control in the months leading up to conception. She has taken folic acid supplements. She has been diabetic since the age of 15 years but has no evidence of diabetic nephropathy or proliferative retinopathy.

What risks, if any, exist for the fetus in a pregnancy such as this in a well-controlled diabetic patient?

The risk for the fetus in diabetic pregnancy is, firstly, congenital abnormality, particularly cardiac, renal and neural tube defects, thought to be related to maternal hyperglycaemia during embryogenesis. This emphasizes the need for good prepregnancy control. Although the risk of fetal abnormality in a well-controlled diabetic is reduced compared with the risk in a poorly controlled diabetic women, it is still important to offer such patients a comprehensive assessment of fetal anatomy by way of a detailed ultrasound scan at 18–20 weeks gestation; this should include an assessment of the fetal heart. In addition, alpha-fetoprotein screening for neural tube defect should be offered at 15–16 weeks gestation. Thus, while

this patient should be reassured that her risk of fetal abnormality is lower than in poorly controlled diabetes, she should still have the reassurance of alpha-fetoprotein testing and ultrasound assessment.

The fetus will also be at risk of macrosomia. Macrosomia is thought to be due to an excess of nutrients such as glucose and free fatty acids being supplied to the fetus, with associated fetal hyperinsulinaemia resulting in increased fetoplacental growth. These fetuses are not simply fat but have increased overall size and organomegaly, particularly of the liver and the heart. Although traditionally macrosomia is associated with poorly controlled diabetes, it is clear that, even where diabetes is optimally controlled throughout the pregnancy, significant macrosomia can still occur. Thus, despite this patient's good control of blood sugar leading up to the pregnancy, and allowing for this to continue throughout the pregnancy, it is still likely that the fetus will be at risk of macrosomia. Macrosomia will place the fetus at risk of obstructed labour and shoulder dystocia. In addition, towards the end of the pregnancy the increased oxygen requirement associated with macrosomia, high insulin levels and consequent glucose metabolism may place the fetus at risk of relative hypoxia. This in turn, can provoke anaerobic metabolism of glucose, acidosis and subsequent fetal compromise. This may be the mechanism behind the feature of 'unexplained' late intrauterine deaths in diabetes, which was considered a problem, at least in the past. Other problems which could place the fetus at risk are miscarriage and premature labour, but, again, these problems are more common if maternal diabetic control is poor.

Intrauterine growth restriction can occur in diabetic pregnancy but this is usually associated with diabetics with extensive microvascular complications, such as diabetic nephropathy and retinopathy. This is therefore unlikely to occur in the present case. Pre-eclampsia is also more common in diabetic pregnancy.

In view of the problems that can occur with regard to fetal growth, it is usual to monitor the fetal growth by ultrasound and well-being by CTG and/or biophysical profile, at least in the third trimester, to anticipate problems and plan delivery.

Outline the medical management of this patient through her pregnancy.

She should continue to aim for optimal glycaemic control through the pregnancy, with blood glucose concentrations of 4–6 mmol/l before meals and less than 7.5 mmol/l postprandially. The target for HbA_{1C} is less than 6% and this should be set before conception. A typical insulin regimen would be use of short-acting insulin before breakfast, lunch and dinner and an intermediate-acting insulin in the evening (Fig. 36.1). Insulin therapy needs to be adjusted and careful records kept of blood glucose and insulin dosage. It is important to provide the patient with a home glucose meter facility for regular and frequent monitoring of her blood sugar, including intermittent nocturnal

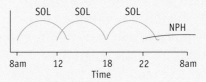

Insulin regimen in pregnancy

- Normally four injections/day
- Omit or change soluble short-acting insulin (SOL) dose as desired
- Basal (bedtime) is usually intermediate-acting insulin (NPH)

Fig. 36.1   *Insulin regimen in pregnancy.*

measurement. It is best if such patients are seen at combined obstetric–diabetic clinics where the obstetric and diabetic problems, which are interlinked, can be reviewed. With regard to insulin requirements, this will require significant adjustment in dose as the pregnancy advances. As hypoglycaemia may occur when the patient is attempting to maintain good control, it is important that both she and her partner are aware of this risk and know how to remedy the situation should it occur, including the use of glucagon. Over the whole of her pregnancy, the increased insulin requirements may be as much as 2 or 3 times that of the prepregnancy requirements. The underlying mechanism behind the increased insulin demand is thought to be, at least in part, due to the secretion of placental hormones such as human placental lactogen, which can act as an insulin antagonist. Regular assessment of her optic fundi is also important to ensure that she does not have proliferative retinopathy.

She attends regularly and maintains good glycaemic control. At 20 weeks gestation a detailed ultrasound scan shows no

evidence of any fetal abnormality. Serum alpha-fetoprotein measurement had previously been normal. She is reassured but 1 week later is referred as an emergency by her general practitioner as she is complaining of rigors and abdominal pain. On examination, she is pyrexial with a temperature of 39°C, her abdomen is tender and she has bilateral renal angle tenderness. What is the likely diagnosis and what implications does it have for the pregnancy?

The likely diagnosis is pyelonephritis. Diabetic mothers are more at risk of urinary tract infection and pyelonephritis. As well as causing an upset in the control of their diabetes, it will also place them at risk of preterm labour. Prompt treatment should be instituted, with intravenous fluids, broad-spectrum antibiotics and analgesia. A diabetic physician should be involved to ensure that her diabetic control is optimal, to avoid the development of problems such as diabetic ketoacidosis, which may be particularly harmful to the fetus.

The pyelonephritis resolves by treatment with a cephalosporin and, despite transient upset in her diabetic control associated with this severe infection, good control is regained within 1 week and she is discharged.

At 30 weeks gestation, in the course of her combined obstetric–diabetic review, you find that her blood pressure is 130/95 mmHg. On rechecking it is 120/90 mmHg. Her booking blood pressure was 110/78 mmHg. What would your concern be and how would you assess the situation?

Pre-eclampsia is more common in diabetic pregnancy and any possible warning sign of superimposed pre-eclampsia should be taken seriously. The patient should have a full assessment of her blood pressure and biochemistry, checking particularly for any increase in uric acid or liver func-

tion test abnormality. Platelet count should also be checked. Such investigations can be carried out on an outpatient basis in a day assessment unit and it is important to establish rapidly whether or not this complication has arisen.

You send her round to the day assessment unit where, over a period of 4 h, her average blood pressure is 126/88 mmHg, biochemistry is entirely normal and there is no evidence of proteinuria. CTG shows a normal reactive pattern in keeping with fetal well-being and you arrange to see her a few days later to ensure that her blood pressure remains normal, which it does.

A series of ultrasound scans between 28 and 36 weeks gestation have demonstrated that the fetus is indeed macrosomic, despite good glycaemic control, with the fetus lying above the 95th centile for gestation in terms of weight as assessed by abdominal circumference. At 36 weeks gestation you discuss delivery with her. She is keen to have a spontaneous labour and delivery, but is conscious that she is at increased risk of caesarean section because of the fetal macrosomia. Regular fetal assessment has shown no evidence of fetal compromise and you plan to continue with twice-weekly assessments until delivery. How should labour be managed?

With regard to the fetus, the main risks in labour are asphyxia and trauma from shoulder dystocia. Where a fetus has an estimated weight of over 4.5 kg it is usual to offer caesarean section in view of the risk of shoulder dystocia in diabetic pregnancy. Continuous monitoring of the fetal heart rate during labour should take place in diabetic pregnancy, and progress in labour should be carefully assessed for evidence of cephalopelvic disproportion and the risk of shoulder dystocia. If there is concern with regard to the possibility of cephalopelvic disproportion, caesarean section should be performed at an early stage. With regard to glycaemic control, it is usual to obtain good control by way of a regimen such as a constant infusion of 5% glucose administered at an initial rate of 100 ml/h in conjunction with intravenous infusion of soluble insulin at an initial dose of 1 unit/h, titrating this against hourly blood glucose measurements. She should also receive prophylactic antibiotics at the time of the caesarean section, if this is necessary.

Frequent variable and late decelerations occur at 3 cm cervical dilatation and you perform a caesarean section for suspected fetal distress The baby is born in good condition. What complications would the baby be at risk of postnatally?

Although infant respiratory distress syndrome is more common in infants of diabetic mothers, at this gestation this is unlikely to be a problem. Transient tachypnoea of the newborn is also more common, particularly if delivery is by caesarean section. In view of the macrosomia, however, the neonate may suffer from problems such as hypoglycaemia, polycythaemia and neonatal jaundice. Thus, careful observation of the fetus is required following delivery.

Should the mother's insulin dose be adjusted after delivery?

Insulin requirements fall to prepregnancy values rapidly following delivery of the placenta and it is usual to re-establish the prepregnancy dose of insulin.

Venous thrombosis

A 27 year old primigravida, who weighs 88 kg and is 1.55 m tall, presents at 11 weeks gestation with a painful swollen left leg. She has been in bed most of the past week with bad morning sickness and has not been able to keep much food or drink down. On taking a family history you find that her mother and her grandmother both had 'clots' in their legs associated with pregnancy.

How would you investigate the leg symptoms?

She has several risk factors for venous thrombosis, including pregnancy, obesity (BMI > 29), hyperemesis (often associated with dehydration and immobility) and a family history of pregnancy-associated thrombosis. It is essential to investigate her for deep venous thrombosis (DVT). The clinical diagnosis of DVT during pregnancy is unreliable, particularly as leg swelling and discomfort are common features of normal pregnancy. Objective diagnosis of DVT in pregnancy is therefore essential, with real-time or duplex ultrasound being the first-line diagnostic test. Failure to identify a DVT will place her life at risk from pulmonary embolism, while unnecessary treatment will expose her not only to anticoagulants, but will also label her as having had a venous thromboembolism (VTE). This will affect her future health care, such as contraception, and thromboprophylaxis in future pregnancies. It is also import-ant to look for any other underlying problem that could cause unilateral leg swelling and pain, such as a ruptured Baker cyst or soft-tissue injury. You should enquire about any symptoms suggestive of pulmonary thromboembolism resulting from a DVT, such as chest pain, breathlessness or haemoptysis.

Duplex and real-time Doppler ultrasound (Fig. 37.1) show occlusive thrombus in the left common femoral vein. Note that almost 90% of gestation-associated DVTs occur on the left side, in contrast to the non-pregnant situation, where only 55% of DVTs occur on the left. This may reflect compression of the left iliac vein by the right iliac artery and the ovarian artery, which cross the vein on the left side only. More than 70% of gestational DVTs are iliofemoral, compared with only around 9% in the non-pregnant. Iliofemoral DVTs are more likely to embolise, and lead to pulmonary thromboembolism, than calf vein thrombosis. This is an important difference between gestational and non-gestational DVT.

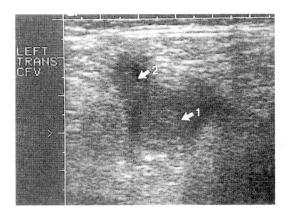

Fig. 37.1   Ultrasound scan of the common femoral vein demonstrating clot in the vessel. Arrow 1: thrombus in the femoral vein; arrow 2: thrombus in the long saphenous vein. (Reproduced with permission of Blackwell Science Ltd.)

Should you screen for thrombophilia?

Many DVTs occurring in young women during the course of pregnancy are the first manifestion of underlying thrombophilic problems. Around 50% of pregnancy-associated VTEs are associated with an identifiable heritable thrombophilia. The most common problem is factor V Leiden. This is the commonest congenital thrombophilia, with a gene frequency of between 3 and 10% in Western populations. Investigations of patients with a DVT in pregnancy may find factor V Leiden in over 20% of cases. Factor V Leiden is an abnormal form of factor V which has a normal coagulation function but which is resistant to breakdown by the inhibitor of coagulation, activated protein C, resulting in an increase in thrombotic risk. It has also been associated with a number of thrombotic problems associated with the oral contraceptive pill. Deficiencies of the endogenous anticoagulants antithrombin, protein C and protein S are much less common than factor V Leiden and, taken together, they will be found in around only 5% of women with a DVT in pregnancy. Antithrombin deficiency carries a very high risk of venous thrombosis in pregnancy. Thromboses that occur in association with protein C and protein S deficiency are more commonly seen postpartum. More recently a variant has been found in the prothrombin gene affecting 2% of western European populations. Heterozygotes for this variant, prothrombin 20210A, have higher levels of prothrombin and enhanced risk of thrombosis. Lupus anticoagulant and anticardiolipin antibodies, the main forms of acquired thrombophilia, can also underlie venous thrombosis in pregnancy. Investigations should therefore be performed, especially in view of the family history, to determine if she has congenital or acquired thrombophilia. If a congenital defect is found or suspected, the family should be investigated. Increasingly, there is evidence to link heritable thrombophilia to pregnancy complications, including miscarriage, IUGR, pre-eclampsia, abruption and fetal loss.

Although the results of a thrombophilia screen will not influence immediate management, it can influence the duration and intensity of anticoagulation, such as in antithrombin deficiency. It is important to be aware of the effects of pregnancy and thrombus on the results of a thrombophilia screen. Protein S levels fall in pregnancy, making it virtually impossible to diagnose protein S deficiency. Activated protein C resistance occurs in around 40% of pregnancies and anticardiolipin antibodies can also influence this test. Antithrombin may be reduced when thrombus is present. Genotyping for factor V Leiden and prothrombin G20210A will not be influenced by pregnancy or current thrombosis. Because of these problems thrombophilia screening is often delayed until after pregnancy and after anticoagulant therapy has ceased.

On investigation she is found to be heterozygous for prothrombin 20210A. How would your treat her?

Treatment of gestational VTE centres on the use of unfractionated heparin (UFH) or low molecular weight heparin (LMWH), owing to the fetal hazards of coumarins (warfarin embryopathy) and haemorrhagic complications for mother and fetus. Neither UFH nor LMWH cross the placenta and thus there is no risk of teratogenesis or fetal haemorrhage. However, prolonged use of UFH can be associated with osteoporosis, allergy and heparin-induced thrombocytopenia. In contrast, LMWHs appear to have a very much lower risk of these complications.

The properties of LMWH allow the use of a fixed-dose, subcutaneous regimen in the acute treatment of VTE, minimizing or avoiding the need for monitoring. Meta-analyses of randomized controlled trials in non-pregnant women have compared LMWH to UFH in the initial treatment of DVT. LMWH was found to be more effective than UFH and was also associated with a lower risk of bleeding complications. Graduated elastic compression stockings should also be employed, together with leg elevation.

In view of the alterations in the pharmacokinetics of LMWH in pregnancy, a twice-daily dosage regimen for these LMWHs in the treatment of VTE in pregnancy has been recommended. One dose regimen for the administration of a LMWH (enoxaparin) in the immediate management of VTE in pregnancy is shown in Table 37.1; the initial dose of enoxaparin (1 mg/kg) is based on the early pregnancy weight, as LMWH does not cross the placenta. Enoxaparin is available in prefilled syringes of 40, 60, 80 and 100 mg. The dose closest to the woman's weight should be employed. Heparin activity can be monitored by measuring the peak anti-Xa activity (3 h postinjection). A suitable target therapeutic range is 0.6–1.2 units/ml. If the peak anti-Xa level is above the upper limit of the therapeutic target range, the dose of LMWH should be reduced (e.g. for enoxaparin 100 mg b.d. to 80 mg b.d.), and peak anti-Xa activity reassessed. In this case the starting dose would be 80 mg enoxaparin twice a day.

Table 37.1 *Initial dose of enoxaparin for acute treatment of VTE*

Early pregnancy weight (kg)	Initial dose of enoxaparin (mg twice daily)
<50	40
50–69	60
70–89	80
≥90	100

The platelet count should be checked 4–8 days after treatment commences, then about once a month, to detect heparin-induced thrombocytopenia, which is associated with further thrombotic complications. Pregnant women who develop heparin-induced thrombocytopenia and require ongoing anticoagulant therapy should be managed with the heparinoid, danaparoid sodium.

Can she be treated as an outpatient?

The patient can be taught to self-inject and can be managed as an outpatient once the acute event is controlled. Arrangements should be made to allow safe disposal of needles and syringes.

How long should she be treated?

The duration of therapeutic anticoagulant treatment for acute VTE in the non-pregnant is usually 6 months. As pregnancy is associated with prothrombotic coagulation changes and reduced venous flow, it is logical to apply this same duration of treatment to gestational VTE. When the VTE occurs early in the pregnancy, then, provided that there are no additional risk factors, the dose of LMWH could be reduced to prophylactic levels (e.g. 40 mg enoxaparin once per day or 5000 iu dalteparin once a day) after 6 months. In this case, in view of the additional risk factors, it may be of value to continue on therapeutic doses until delivery is planned. After delivery, treatment should continue for at least 6–12 weeks. Warfarin can be used following delivery. If she chooses to commence warfarin postpartum, this can be started on the second or third postnatal day. The INR should be maintained between 2.0 and 3.0. LMWH treatment should be continued until the INR is > 2.0 on two successive days.

Induction of labour is planned at term: how would you adjust her LMWH treatment?

The dose of heparin should be reduced to a thromboprophylactic level (40 mg enoxaparin or 5000 iu dalteparin once daily) on the day before delivery and omitted on the morning of planned delivery to allow epidural anaesthesia. Graduated elastic compression stockings can be worn during labour. The treatment dose can be recommenced after delivery. If she wishes an epidural anaesthetic for pain relief, this should not be employed until at least 12 h after the previous prophylactic dose of LMWH, and LMWH should not be given for at least 3 h after the epidural catheter has been removed. These precautions minimize the very small risk of epidural haematoma.

Is she at risk of post-thrombotic syndrome?

Yes, 80% of women with VTE develop post-thrombotic syndrome, and over 60% will have objectively confirmed deep venous insufficiency following a treated DVT.

Intrauterine growth restriction

A 35 year old primigravida attends the antenatal clinic at 32 weeks gestation. The symphyseal–fundal height is 27 cm.

How would you manage the case?

The uterine size is small for the gestation, raising concern for fetal growth. The small-for-dates fetus carries an increased risk of intrauterine death, intrapartum asphyxia, neonatal hypoglycaemia and possible long-term neurological impairment. The perinatal mortality is also higher: > 10th centile overall 12:1000, 5th–10th centile 22:1000, < 5th centile 190:1000 (80% occur in utero, with 50% of these occurring after 36 weeks). Thus, the main concern in this case is that the fetus is suffering from intrauterine growth restriction (IUGR). This is a term that should be used for those fetuses where there is clear evidence that growth has been impaired. It can only be confirmed by studying the rate of growth over time and therefore requires serial ultrasound assessments. It is important to appreciate the difference between a small-for-dates and growth-restricted (IUGR) fetus. A small-for-gestational-age (SGA) fetus is one where the weight is < 10th centile for gestational age. These fetuses may simply be inherently small, but healthy and growing along their centile. In contrast, IUGR refers to any fetus failing to achieve its growth potential. Not all small-for-dates fetuses are growth restricted and not all growth-restricted

fetuses are small for dates. Clearly it is essential to check that the gestational age is accurate in order to make the diagnosis.

Intrauterine growth restriction is usually classified as symmetrical or asymmetrical. In the former, the head size and trunk are reduced, concomitantly. The vast majority of these symmetrically small fetuses will represent the lower end of the normal range for size. However, particularly in those that are very small, antenatal problems such as intrauterine infection or a congenital abnormality may be present. Thus, ultrasound should be used to check for any structural abnormality. Asymmetrical IUGR is more commonly encountered. This reflects an inadequate supply of nutrition to the baby due to inadequate placental invasion of the maternal circulation and/or placental infarction. In response to this placental problem, the fetus will redistribute its blood flow to ensure that the brain, heart and adrenal glands are preserved in their function, with less blood flow going to the liver and kidneys. As a consequence of this, growth of the trunk and, in particular, the abdominal girth, which includes the abdominal fat stores and liver glycogen stores, will fall disproportionately to the head — the so-called brain sparing effect. While asymmetrical IUGR can occur on its own, it is often linked to pre-eclampsia.

There are many factors associated with an increased risk of IUGR. These include maternal factors, such as chronic hypertension or connective tissue disease, smoking, poor nutrition, age < 16 or > 35 years at the time of delivery, and social deprivation. Fetoplacental factors relating to IUGR include intrauterine infection and chromosomal abnormalities.

Screening for IUGR with clinical techniques such as estimation of the symphyseal–fundal height is a routine part of antenatal care. Where there is a suspicion that the baby may be small for dates, it is important to confirm this by ultrasound. Thus, the woman should be referred for ultrasound scan to assess fetal growth and liquor volume. A single ultrasound scan in the third trimester cannot differentiate between a baby that is small for gestational age and one that is suffering from IUGR. Thus, serial scans are required. The best single discriminator of fetal weight is the abdominal circumference.

Ultrasound scan shows that the abdominal circumferemce is just above the 5th centile, whereas the head circumference is on the 20th centile. What further investigations are warranted?

The low abdominal circumference and its disproportion to the head circumference suggests that this fetus may suffer from IUGR. Serial ultrasound scans should be performed to study growth at fortnightly intervals. It is also important to look for additional evidence of placental insufficiency, such as reduced liquor volume or an abnormal umbilical artery Doppler flow velocity waveform. As there are many conditions that can underlie IUGR, the obstetrician should also consider whether any such conditions are present and investigate as appropriate; such investigations might include measurement of anticardiolipin antibodies, which are associated with thrombotic problems, placental damage and pregnancy complications including IUGR, pre-eclampsia and miscarriage. It is also important to identify whether the fetus is compromised, as this would lead to delivery; this is usually assessed either by way of a biophysical profile (Fig. 38.1) or with CTG, the latter ideally coupled with an assessment of liquor volume. Where there is clear evidence of growth restriction, such monitoring of fetal well-being is usually carried out on a twice-weekly basis. There is no proven medical intervention in late-onset IUGR; however, if preterm delivery is considered a possibility, the patient should receive steroids to enhance fetal lung maturation.

At the next assessment 2 weeks later, the abdominal circumference is crossing the 5th centile, but head growth appears to be continuing. Biophysical profiles show normal fetal movement patterns but reduced liquor volume. However, the Doppler flow velocity waveform of the umbilical artery shows absent end-diastolic flow. How would you manage the situation?

In the situation of IUGR (Fig. 38.2) in the 3rd trimester with an abnormal umbilical artery flow velocity waveform, there are two options. The first would be to proceed to delivery, as the fetus will be at high risk. The alternative is to continue with intensive fetal surveillance with a view to delivery, usually by caesarean section, should there be evidence of stress, such as an abnormal CTG or biophysical profile.

The biophysical profile

		Score
Nonstress test	Reactive is two or more fetal heart rate accelerations in a 20-min period	2
	Nonreactive is none or one fetal heart rate acceleration	0
Fetal breathing movements	One episode of prolonged breathing (>60 s) within 30 min	2
	Fetal breathing movement absent	0
Gross fetal body movements, i.e. movements of the trunk	Fetal movements present with a minimum of three movements within a 30-min period	2
	Fetal movements absent or reduced	0
Fetal tone, i.e. limb flexion and extension	Normal: one episode of limb flexion and extension	2
	Abnormal: extremities extended with no return to flexion	0
Amniotic fluid volume	Normal: largest pocket of fluid is >1cm in vertical diameter in a cord-free pool*	2
	Decreased liquor volume	0
		Total score = 0–10

*Many obstetricians prefer to use a greater limit than 1cm in assessing liquor volume and many use a cut off of 2 or 3cm.
Alternatively, the amniotic fluid index, derived from measuring fluid volume in four quadrants of the uterus, can be used.

Fig. 38.1   *The biophysical profile.*

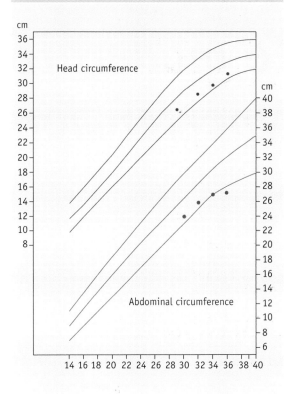

**Growth chart showing IUGR
with relative head-sparing**

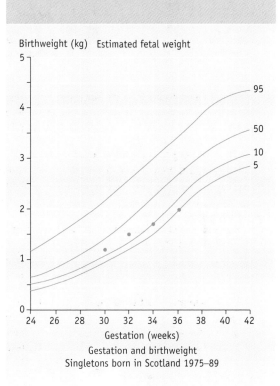

Estimated fetal weight

(a)

(b)

Fig. 38.2 *Growth chart showing IUGR with relative head-sparing. Note the fall-off in abdominal circumference growth. Liquor volume was reduced, although the CTG was satisfactory. The patient was delivered at 36+ weeks and the baby weighed 2.1 kg. The placenta was infarcted.*

Mild to moderate hypertension

A 25 year old nulliparous patient is found to have a diastolic blood pressure of 95 mmHg at 32 weeks gestation. Her blood pressure recording at 9 weeks gestation was 115/78 mmHg.

How would you assess the situation further?

The main concern here is that she is developing pre-eclampsia. Pre-eclampsia is a multisystem disorder of unknown aetiology peculiar to pregnancy. It is characterized clinically by hypertension, proteinuria and often fluid retention, but can appear in a variety of presentations due to the multisystem nature of the disease process. The underlying pathophysiology is widespread endothelial damage and dysfunction mediated by a variety of mechanisms, including proinflammatory cytokines and leucocyte activation, platelet and coagulation activation, and disturbed lipid metabolism. This is associated with increased vascular reactivity, reduced maternal plasma volume and increased vascular permeability. Activation of the coagulation system can progress in severe cases to disseminated intravascular coagulation. There is damage and dysfunction of the kidney, where tubular dysfunction leads to high levels of uric acid in the plasma and glomerular damage results in proteinuria. Liver dysfunction, cardiac failure, pulmonary oedema, central nervous system problems (eclampsia, intracerebral haemorrhage) and adverse fetal effects due to placental insufficiency and iatrogenic preterm delivery also occur. It is an extremely variable and unpredictable condition and progression is often more rapid the earlier in pregnancy it occurs. Delivery will result in disease regression. The purpose of antenatal screening is to identify women developing the problem and prevent both the maternal complications (cerebral injury, multisystem failure) and fetal complications (IUGR, intrauterine death and abruption) of severe disease by timely delivery of the baby.

Mild to moderate hypertension is usually identified when diastolic blood pressure is between 90 and 110 mmHg in the absence of proteinuria. These women should have a repeat blood pressure measurement ≥4 h later. If high blood pressure is confirmed, basic surveillance of twice-weekly monitoring of blood pressure and urine for protein, as well as clinical assessment of maternal and fetal well-being, is required.

It would be useful to obtain a full blood count, urea and electrolytes and urate in the first instance. Enhanced surveillance is required if the diastolic blood pressure is > 100 mmHg at < 37 weeks gestation, or there is a blood pressure increment of > 25 mmHg over the booking blood pressure. Enhanced surveillance is also required if there is clinical evidence of IUGR, concern over maternal or fetal well-being or abnormal biochemistry. When such situations arise, it is usual to proceed to thrice-weekly assessments of blood pressure, urinalysis and full blood count, together with urea and electrolytes, urate and liver function tests. In addition, the fetus should also be assessed with an ultrasound scan to determine fetal growth and a CTG or biophysical profile to monitor fetal well-being.

There is no indication for admission or bed rest in women with mild to moderate hypertension unless there are further abnormalities such as significant fetal compromise or abnormal biochemistry, for example, significantly abnormal liver function tests or evidence of other complications, such as HELLP syndrome, developing. (HELLP syndrome is an acronym for *h*aemolysis, *e*levated *l*iver enzymes and *l*ow *p*latelets — a severe form of pre-eclampsia with serious liver involvement and where hypertension itself may not be severe). Thus, antenatal care for patients with mild to moderate disease can usually be managed effectively, both clinically and in terms of cost, through a day-care unit or in the community. The value of anti-hypertensive therapy in these women is not clear. Meta-analyses suggest that it leads to a reduction in the development of proteinuric disease, severe high blood pressure and respiratory distress in the fetus, but there is no benefit in terms of gestation at delivery or obstetric intervention. Thus, perhaps antihypertensive therapy should be reserved for those with early-onset disease, i.e. < 32 weeks gestation, or those with a diastolic blood pressure > 100 mmHg, although the reduction in proteinuria and severe hypertension may be of value in reducing the perceived need for intervention such as early delivery. If an antihypertensive agent is to be prescribed, the most commonly used ones in the United Kingdom are perhaps methyldopa and labetalol. Where a second-line agent is required, nifedipine can be employed.

With regard to the drugs used, methyldopa is the most extensively studied drug in the treatment of hypertension in pregnancy. Although it is no longer commonly used other than in problem pregnancies, its safety profile and efficacy have allowed it to maintain its position in obstetric care. While effective in blood pressure control, one drawback in the use of methyldopa is the frequency of side-effects, which can affect up to 15% of patients. There are also good data on methyldopa with regard to long-term follow-up of children, which has shown no long-term adverse effect. With regard to adrenoceptor antagonists, the only agents that have been studied extensively in pregnancy are atenolol, labetalol and oxprenolol. These agents are often preferred to methyldopa by obstetricians because of the low incidence of side-effects. They are all highly effective as first-line antihypertensive agents and do not appear to affect adversely fetal monitoring tests, in particular, CTG. Long-term use of adrenoceptor antagonists has been associated with an increased risk of growth restriction, particularly with atenolol, but more recent data suggest that this is a non-specific effect of antihypertensive therapy, as opposed to a specific effect of adrenoceptor antagonists. In short term use in the third trimester, for patients with mild to moderate disease, this does not appear to be a significant clinical problem.

It should also be noted that these women are at increased risk of chronic hypertension in later life and, should the hypertension persist after delivery, investigations should be carried out to look for an underlying medical cause.

Severe hypertension

An 18 year old para 0+1 presents at 26 weeks gestation feeling slightly nauseated, with a blood pressure of 165/105 mmHg and proteinuria ++ on dipstick testing. At booking her blood pressure was 140/90 mmHg and it transpires that, as a child, she was frequently admitted to hospital for urinary tract infections. She presents with her boyfriend, who has been drinking, and they are both keen to get away as soon as possible for a party.

What is the differential diagnosis?

- Pre-eclampsia
- Renal impairment following recurrent urinary tract infections
- Essential hypertension and coincidental urinary tract infection.

What is the initial management of this couple?

It is essential to stress the importance of these findings to the couple and to advise that they cancel the plans for the party. Admission is highly appropriate as pre-eclampsia presenting in the very preterm is often severe. The blood pressure should be repeated and further maternal assessment made by enquiry about headache or flashing lights (pre-eclampsia), epigastric pain (HELLP syn-drome), dysuria (urinary infection) and past history of any renal follow-up or investigation. Blood should be sent for urate (rises in pre-eclampsia), platelets (falls in pre-eclampsia and HELLP syndrome) and liver function tests (again for HELLP syndrome).

Fetal assessment clinically and with ultrasound is important, looking for evidence of IUGR, reduced liquor volume or reduced end-diastolic flow in the umbilical artery.

What do you think is the most likely diagnosis?

It seems too coincidental for essential hypertension and urinary tract infection to occur simultaneously — a single pathology is more likely. It may be difficult to tease renal impairment from pre-eclampsia, although an ultrasound of the kidneys may show scarring following the repeated infections. Renal impairment will in any case predispose to pre-eclampsia, and in practice it should be assumed that this is pre-eclampsia and management planned accordingly.

Pre-eclampsia is said to be a multisystem disorder. Which systems can be affected?

There is reduced maternal plasma volume and increased vascular permeability, some degree of intravascular coagulopathy (may lead to DIC), glomerular damage (leading to proteinuria), liver dysfunction (see HELLP syndrome below), cardiac failure, pulmonary oedema, central nervous system problems (eclampsia, haemorrhage) and adverse fetal effects. It is an extremely variable and unpredictable condition. The purpose of antenatal screening is to prevent both the maternal complications (cerebral injury, multisystem failure) and fetal complications (IUGR, intrauterine death and abruption) of severe disease by timely delivery of the baby.

What is the management plan?

The aim is to prolong pregnancy further, to give the baby a better chance of survival, delivering before either the mother or baby deteriorate. The mother should have a urine output chart (minimum 600 ml/day), daily urea and electrolytes, urate, platelets and liver function tests and be asked to report any deterioration of symptoms. She should be given steroids (to enhance fetal lung maturity) as preterm delivery is very likely and the baby should be scanned every few days for a biophysical profile (particularly liquor volume) and Doppler flow studies. If either mother or baby deteriorate significantly, then delivery is indicated.

Treatment of the mother with antihypertensives masks the sign of hypertension but does not alter the course of the disease, although it may allow prolongation of the pregnancy and thereby improve fetal outcome. Oral methyldopa and labetolol are commonly used as first-line agents, and oral nifedipine as a second-line agent.

Ergometrine (including Syntometrine®) should not be used for the third stage as it may exacerbate hypertension. Syntocinon® 10 units i.m. or i.v. stat should be given instead.

What is HELLP syndrome?

This is an acronym for haemolysis, elevated liver enzymes (particularly transaminases) and low platelets. It is a variant of pre-eclampsia affecting 4–12% of those with pre-eclampsia/eclampsia and is commoner in multigravidae. There may be epigastric pain, nausea, vomiting and right upper quadrant tenderness. Aspartate aminotransferase (AST) rises first (> 48 i.u./l) then lactate dehydrogenase (LDH) (> 164 i.u./l). An LDH > 600 i.u./l level indicates severe disease. Hypertension may not be severe. A blood film may show burr cells and polychromasia consistent with haemolysis, although anaemia is uncommon. There may also be acute renal failure and DIC, and there is an increased incidence of abruption. There is also an increased incidence (although still rare) of hepatic haematoma and hepatic rupture, leading to profuse intraperitoneal bleeding. It can progress to multiorgan failure with adult respiratory distress syndrome. HELLP is a life-threatening condition. Management is to stabilize coagulation, assess fetal well-being and usually to proceed to urgent delivery, as in pre-eclampsia. There is evidence that high-dose steroid therapy may reduce the extent of the liver damage and hasten postpartum hepatic recovery.

Three days after admission her blood pressure is persistently 170/110 mmHg despite oral labetolol (severe hypertension is defined as a single diastolic blood pressure >120 mmHg on any one occasion or >110 mmHg on two occasions ≥ 4 h apart). Having seemed relatively well, she suddenly starts fitting. What is happening and what should be done?

This is an eclamptic seizure. Management is as follows:

- Turn her onto her side to avoid aortocaval compression.
- Insert an airway and give high-flow oxygen, e.g. 6 l/min.
- Give 4 g magnesium sulphate over 10–15 min i.v., or i.m. if access is not possible. This is significantly more effective than phenytoin or diazepam in preventing further convulsions. Although magnesium sulphate is not sedative, it can depress neuromuscular transmission (reversed with calcium gluconate). Reduced patellar reflexes usually precede respiratory depression.
- Consider paralysis and ventilation if the fits are prolonged or recurrent.
- Consider urgent delivery by caesarean section.
- Set up an intravenous infusion of magnesium sulphate.

The aim is then to reduce diastolic blood pressure to < 100 mmHg, prevent pulmonary oedema, prevent convulsions and maintain the urine output:

- Involve senior obstetric and anaesthetic staff.
- Monitor the blood pressure and adjust antihypertensives accordingly (e.g. i.v. labetolol or hydralazine).
- Monitor the Sao_2 and arrange a chest X-ray if the saturation drops below 93% or there is cough, dyspnoea or tachypnoea.
- Catheterize and measure hourly urine volumes. Central monitoring with a CVP or Swan–Ganz catheter will be useful in differentiating the oliguria of intravascular depletion from the oliguria of renal failure. This will be even more relevant if there has been a large blood loss at caesarean section.

Patients with pulmonary oedema and adult respiratory distress syndrome may require ventilation, and dialysis support may be necessary if acute renal failure develops.

She is delivered of a baby girl weighing 600 g who makes good progress. The mother herself has one further convulsion, but goes on to make a good recovery. Can eclampsia be prevented in her next pregnancy?

The hypertensive diseases of pregnancy tend to be less severe with each subsequent pregnancy to the same partner provided that there is no underlying medical condition, such as SLE or essential hypertension. Where such an underlying problem exists, the risk of recurrence is much greater. In view of the severity of her pre-eclampsia and its early onset, she remains at high risk and should receive intensive antenatal monitoring. There is some evidence that low-dose aspirin taken from early pregnancy (< 17 weeks and probably from the end of the first trimester) may reduce the incidence of IUGR and perinatal mortality in those with previous severe disease. Haemorrhagic problems do not seem to be a cause of clinical difficulty, despite the moderate prolongation of bleeding time, and there is no evidence of any adverse fetal outcome with low-dose aspirin.

Reduced fetal movements

A 28 year old para 1+0 presents at 31 weeks gestation with a 2 day history of reduced fetal movements. She has had a stillbirth in her last pregnancy, but has been keeping well to date on this occasion. When she comes in she is tearful and upset, worried that the baby's kicks are not as strong.

What are the possible underlying reasons for her concern?

It is quite possible that she is worried that her baby has died, particularly as she may have felt reduced fetal movements prior to her previous stillbirth. Assuming the baby is alive, however, the reduced movements may indicate that the baby is becoming compromised and that closer monitoring or delivery is required. It is more likely, however, that the baby is well and that the reduced movement is within physiologically normal limits. Indeed it could also be that the movements themselves have not changed but that she has been too busy to notice them.

Reduction or cessation of fetal movement may precede fetal death by up to a day or even more. Not all fetal deaths, however, are necessarily preventable by this knowledge: some are not preceded by a reduction in movements, and for others the fetal death may occur too quickly after the reduction in movement to take any useful action. Nonetheless, the symptom is an important one and should be taken seriously.

What further background information would you wish to elicit?

It is important to explore the history of her previous pregnancy. Was any cause ever identified for the stillbirth, e.g. pre-eclampsia, abruption, IUGR, antiphospholipid syndrome, infection, structural or chromosomal abnormality? At what gestation did it occur? (If it was at 32 weeks maternal anxiety at 31 weeks gestation in this pregnancy would be particularly understandable.) Have any steps been taken in this pregnancy to exclude a recurrent cause, e.g. amniocentesis for a chromosomal abnormality, serial ultrasound growth measurements for growth restriction, blood pressure checks for pre-eclampsia, or a detailed anatomy scan looking for structural abnormalities? Was the maternal serum alpha-fetoprotein at 16 weeks elevated? (This is a marker for a poorer fetal outcome even in the presence of a normal anatomy scan.)

In this case, the previous stillbirth had been at 33 weeks gestation and the patient had presented after not feeling any movement for 5 days.

The baby had been small (just below the 10th centile for gestation) and postmortem examination had shown bilateral renal agenesis (Potter syndrome), which is incompatible with postnatal survival because of associated pulmonary hypoplasia. She had been advised that the recurrence risk was small, and at 18 weeks in this pregnancy she had had a detailed scan which had shown that both kidneys were present, the bladder filled well and there was a normal volume of liquor around the baby.

It is therefore most unlikely that her previous obstetric history would have any direct bearing on reduced movements at 31 weeks in this pregnancy and attention should be focused on the more recent history.

What features of the history and examination would you be interested in, and what investigations would you organize?

Are there any underlying medical problems that might put this pregnancy at increased risk (e.g. diabetes mellitus, renal impairment, connective tissue disorder or severe hypertension), or has there been any history of trauma (increased risk of placental abruption or spontaneous fetomaternal haemorrhage)? Has she been keeping well, or has there been any pain (to suggest abruption), headache or blurred vision (to suggest pregnancy-induced hypertension) or fever (to suggest infection, for example of the urinary tract)? Have there been any symptoms or signs of labour (show, contractions or ruptured membranes)?

Check pulse, blood pressure and urinalysis. She may be distressed and hypotensive in abruption, and the uterus would classically feel hard and tender. Fetal lie, presentation and growth should be assessed by palpation (growth restricted fetuses are more at risk of compromise), and then the fetal heart auscultated. While this may be achieved using a Pinard, the use of CTG or portable Doppler probe has the advantage that the parents can also hear the fetal heartbeat and are more reassured.

Thereafter a CTG tracing should be continued, ensuring that:

- The baseline is between 110 and 150 b.p.m.
- There is good variability (5–15 b.p.m.)
- There are accelerations (of 15 b.p.m. and lasting longer than 15 s).
- There are no variable or late decelerations.

If this is normal, the growth is clinically satisfactory and the mother is feeling some movements again, it is probably reasonable to reassure her and arrange an appointment for the next clinic. It is often helpful to offer her a 'kick chart' (Fig. 41.1), so that she can record the movements on a daily basis and refer herself again if there are further reductions. If, however, there is any other reason for concern (and the anxiety about the previous stillbirth might be a valid reason in itself), it is important to take investigations further in the form of ultrasound assessment.

The ultrasonographer should measure fetal growth (to exclude growth restriction) and perform a 'biophysical profile' to further assess fetal well-being. The finding of all four of the parameters below is reassuring.

Fetal breathing	Lasting more than 30 s in 30 min
Fetal movements	More than three limb or trunk movements in 30 min
Fetal tone	One return to flexion (of neck) after extension, or one hand opening and closing
Liquor	More than 3 cm depth in two planes

Further assessment can be made using Doppler studies of the umbilical artery. This gives an indication of downstream vascular resistance in the placenta by examining flow velocity waveforms. Loss of blood flow at the end of diastole suggests placental ischaemia. Absent end-diastolic flow (Fig. 41.2) is associated with a high perinatal mortality and

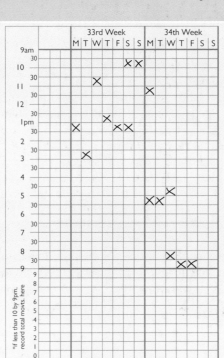

Fig. 41.1 The Cardiff 'count-to-ten' fetal activity kick chart. The mother is asked to start counting movements from 0900, and to note the time each day that 10 movements have been felt. If, by 2100, there are fewer than 10 movements, she is asked to note the number. If there are fewer than 10 movements on two consecutive days, she is asked to contact her midwife.

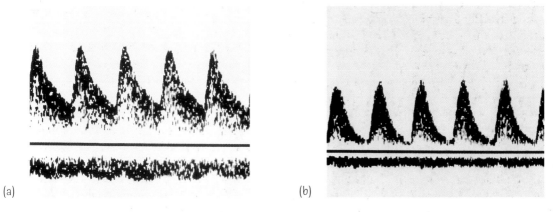

Fig. 41.2 (a) Normal and (b) reduced end-diastolic flow.

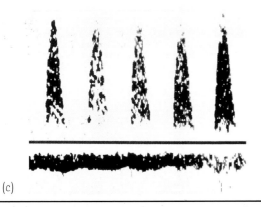

(c)

Fig. 41.2 *(c) Absent end-diastolic flow.*

probably precedes abnormalities in CTGs. Reversed end-diastolic flow carries an even graver prognosis. A normal Doppler is reassuring.

It is obvious that any other identified abnormality (e.g. abruption, growth restriction, pre-eclampsia or fetal abnormality) should be fully investigated and managed.

What advice would you wish to give the mother?

Despite these reassurances, it is to important emphasize that she should return for further monitoring should she feel the movements have again decreased.

Twins

A 41 year old para 0+1 with a 10 year history of infertility is considering sterilization, so that she can 'move forward' with her life, when she finds that she is pregnant. She has had a left salpingectomy for a tubal pregnancy and is aware that she has an increased risk of this also being a tubal pregnancy. A scan is therefore arranged for 6 weeks gestation to confirm that the pregnancy is intrauterine. To her surprise, she finds that she is having twins.

What else would you look for at this scan?

It is important to assess whether this is a mono-chorionic or dichorionic pregnancy (Fig. 42.1) i.e. whether the twins have the same placenta or share a different placenta. Not only do monochorionic pregnancies carry a greater risk of complication than dichorionic, but there are also implications for prenatal diagnosis and antenatal monitoring. Dichorionic twins are much the commoner.

All dizygous (from two eggs) pregnancies are dichorionic, and have separate chorions and amnions. The placental tissue may appear to be continuous but there are no significant vascular communications between the fetuses. Mono-zygotic pregnancies (from the same egg) may also be dichorionic, but may be monochorionic diamniotic or monochorionic monoamniotic (Table 42.1).

Chorionicity is most easily determined in the first or early second trimester:

- Widely separated first trimester sacs or separate placentae are dichorionic.

Table 42.1 *Chorionicity in monozygous twins*

Chorionicity	Frequency (%)	Separation of embryo occurs at (days):
Dichorionic diamniotic	30	<4
Monochorionic diamniotic	66	4–7
Monochorionic monoamniotic	3	7–14
Conjoined	<1	>14

Chorionicity in monozygotic pregnancies

a   b

c   d

Fig. 42.1   *Chorionicity. (a) and (b) Dichorionic diamniotic; (c) monochorionic diamniotic; (d) monochorionic monoamniotic.*

- Those with a 'lambda' or twin-peak' sign at the membrane insertion are dichorionic (Figs 42.2, 42.3).
- Those with a dividing membrane >2 mm are often dichorionic.
- Different sex twins are always dichorionic (and dizygous!).

The twins are dichorionic. How would you counsel her?

In reality, she will be unlikely to take in much useful information at the first visit, as she will be so overwhelmed with the news. She should be seen again in a few weeks' time, but made aware that a proportion of twin pregnancies diagnosed at this early stage are only singletons by the end of the first trimester.

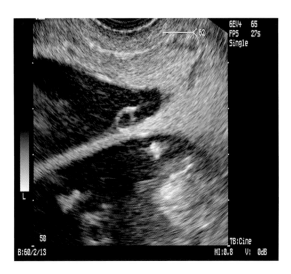

Fig. 42.2   *'Lambda' or 'twin peak' sign of dichorionic pregnancies.*

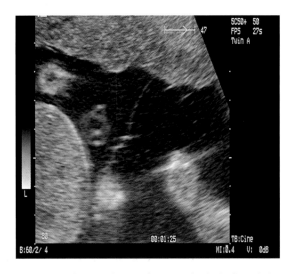

Fig. 42.3   *Thin membrane of a monochorionic diamniotic pregnancy with no 'lambda' sign at insertion.*

At the repeat visit it would be important to discuss whether she wished to consider screening for fetal abnormality. The incidence of fetal abnormality is no different per fetus in a dichorionic pregnancy compared with a singleton pregnancy, although it would have been slightly greater had they been monochorionic.

Structural defects

These are usually confined to one twin (i.e. non-concordant); for example, if there is a neural tube defect in one twin, the other twin is normal in 85–90% of cases. All multiple pregnancies should be offered a detailed midtrimester ultrasound scan. If a major abnormality is found, selective termination with intracardiac potassium chloride is possible in dichorionic pregnancies only, and is most safely carried out before 16–20 weeks (the vascular connection of a monochorionic pregnancy would allow potassium chloride to cross to the other twin).

Chromosomal abnormalities

These are usually non-concordant in dizygotic twins and usually concordant in monozygotic twins. Nuchal translucency measurement at 11–14 weeks is probably more appropriate than serum screening for multiple pregnancies. Two amniocenteses are required in dichorionic pregnancies (very great care must be taken to document which sample has come from which sac).

Her risk of Down syndrome at the age of 41 years is approximately 1:90 per twin. In view of the difficulty she has had in conceiving, however, she may not wish to consider amniocentesis at all.

She opts for nuchal translucency measurements and is reassured by a low risk for both twins. How would you manage the rest of the pregnancy?

As already mentioned, arrange a detailed scan for around 18 weeks to look for evidence of any structural abnormality. Further scans on a 2–4-weekly basis from 24 weeks onwards for growth would then be appropriate (the average weight for twins is 10% lighter than singletons). During antenatal care it should be borne in mind that those with multiple pregnancies are at increased risk of pre-eclampsia. Additional risk factors for pre-eclampsia are that she is a primigravida and older.

At 30 weeks, it is noticed that twin I is smaller than twin II. She has read about twin–twin transfusion sequence and wonders if this might be the problem. What is twin–twin transfusion sequence and could she be correct?

With twin–twin transfusion sequence there is a net flow of blood from one twin to the other through joined placental vasculature. The recipient develops polyhydramnios with raised amniotic pressure, while the donor develops oliguria, oligohydramnios and growth restriction (Fig. 42.4). As she has

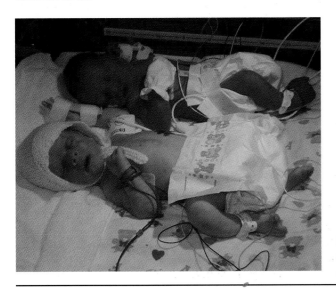

Fig. 42.4 Twin–twin transfusion. The near twin was anaemic at birth with a haemoglobin of 9.7 g/dl. The other was polcythaemic, at 19.1 g/dl.

a dichorionic pregnancy, in which there are no vascular connections, she could not have twin–twin transfusion sequence.

Despite monitoring with CTGs and Doppler flow studies, twin I is found to have no fetal heartbeat at 31 weeks. How does this affect management?

Clearly this will be a devastating blow, mixing grief reactions with the hope of a successful singleton birth. Loss of one twin in the late second or third trimester commonly precipitates labour and 90% will have delivered within 3 weeks. The prognosis for a surviving dichorionic twin is then influenced primarily by its gestation. When a monochorionic twin dies in utero, however, there are additional risks of death (approximately 20%) or cerebral damage (approximately 25%) in the co-twin.

Both twins are cephalic. At 34 weeks she establishes in labour. How would you manage the labour?

In general with twins, providing the first twin is cephalic, evidence would suggest that a trial of labour is appropriate, rather than caesarean section.

Intravenous access should be obtained and blood sent for group and save. An epidural may be very useful in assisting the delivery of a second twin.

The first stage is managed as for singleton pregnancies. Twin I is often monitored with a fetal scalp electrode, although this is clearly not required in this case as the baby is dead. Twin II is monitored abdominally by a CTG. An experienced obstetrician, anaesthetist, paediatricians and two midwives should be present for delivery and an oxytocin infusion should be ready in case uterine activity falls away after delivery of the first twin.

This first twin is delivered as for a singleton. After delivery of the first twin it is often helpful to have someone 'stabilize' the second twin by abdominal palpation to keep the presentation cephalic while a vaginal examinaiton is performed to assess the station of the presenting part. If a second bag of membranes is present, it should not be broken until the presenting part has descended into the pelvis. If twin II lies transverse after the delivery of twin I, external cephalic or breech version may be appropriate. If still transverse (particularly likely if the back is towards the fundus), the choice is between breech extraction (gentle continuous traction on one or both feet through intact membranes) or caesarean section.

It should be remembered that there is an increased incidence of postpartum haemorrhage in multiple pregnancies.

Patient with a previous stillbirth

A 30 year old para 1+0 presents at 12 weeks gestation. She has had a stillbirth 2 years previously, having self-referred to the labour ward at 33 weeks gestation with reduced fetal movements. There was no fetal heart activity on ultrasound scan. Labour was induced and she delivered a stillborn 2.1 kg female baby.

What further information do you need before planning this pregnancy?

It is essential to establish whether any cause was found for the previous stillbirth. A useful obstetric classification is shown in Table 43.1. Was there any evidence of abruption at the time of delivery?

Was a postmortem examination carried out? Or a karyotype of the baby? Were bloods sent for blood grouping and antibodies? Was a HbA_{1C} or random glucose checked? Was there any evidence of congenital infection with toxoplasmosis, rubella, cytomegalovirus or listeria?

Table 43.1 *Obstetrical classification of stillbirth*

Classification	Notes
Congenital anomaly	Any structural or genetic cause
Isoimmunization	Rhesus or non-rhesus
Hypertension of pregnancy	
Antepartum haemorrhage	Abruption and placenta praevia
Trauma/mechanical	e.g. Uterine rupture, birth trauma, cord prolapse
Maternal disorder	e.g. Trauma, diabetes
Miscellaneous	
Unexplained <2500 g	
Unexplained ≥2500 g	

It is also worth noting whether lupus anticoagulant and antiphospholipid antibodies were checked. These are associated with recurrent miscarriage, stillbirth, arterial and venous thrombosis, IUGR, pre-eclampsia and thrombocytopenia. Fifteen per cent of women with a history of recurrent miscarriage (three or more consecutive pregnancy losses) have persistently positive results for phospholipid antibodies and have a rate of fetal loss of 90% when untreated. There is now good evidence that giving low-dose aspirin and subcutaneous heparin throughout pregnancy increases the incidence of live births. The lupus anticoagulant is present in only 5–15% of patients with SLE.

In this instance, the postmortem was negative and the above blood tests were all normal. The classification is therefore in the 'Unexplained <2500 g' category. In general, what congenital anomalies have been associated with perinatal death and how might they be excluded in any subsequent pregnancy?

This is illustrated in Table 43.2. The list is illustrative and not exhaustive.

In view of the fact that the previous stillbirth was unexplained, how would you manage this pregnancy?

The parents are likely to be extremely anxious about the prospects for success this time around, and the anxiety is likely to get worse as 33 weeks approaches. The chance of stillbirth again are low, probably less than 5%, and the couple should be reassured about this. The loss of their daughter should be acknowledged, ideally using her name if she was given one.

In the absence of any identifiable cause, however, it is going to be difficult to monitor for problems. Screening for chromosomal abnormalities and carrying out an ultrasound scan for structural abnormality is likely to provide reassurance, but it is also likely that both of these would have been normal first time around as well. More frequent antenatal visits may also provide reassurance, particularly with growth scans every few weeks from 24 weeks onwards and it would also be relevant to check the liquor volume and umbilical artery Doppler flow.

Throughout, it is important to offer easy access at times of anxiety, particularly if she is worried about fetal movements. The parents should be aware of their point of contact at any time if anxieties occur.

At what stage would you consider delivery?

By 38–39 weeks, many patients will be extremely anxious indeed, and are often keen for labour to be induced. Induction carries the risks of fetal distress and hyperstimulation. Conservative management carries the risk, albeit small, of further in utero demise. The pros and cons of these two should be discussed with the patient to reach an informed decision. The fact that she has already delivered vaginally makes induction rather more likely to succeed, and induction at this stage would not be an unreasonable course of action.

Table 43.2 Congenital anomaly by systems

System	Examples	Diagnosis
CNS	Anencephaly	Ultrasound scan
Cardiovascular	Ventricular hypoplasia, valvular incompetence and arrhythmias	Ultrasound scan
Renal	Infantile polycystic kidney disease, posterior urethral valves, Potter syndrome	Ultrasound scan
Alimentary	Diaphragmatic hernia	Ultrasound scan
Chromosomal	Turner syndrome (45, XO), Down syndrome (47 + 21), Edward syndrome (47 + 18) and Patau syndrome (47 + 13)	While around two-thirds of fetuses with Down syndrome will look normal at 18 weeks, most fetuses with Edward and Patau syndromes do show some abnormality, even though these are often not specific or diagnostic. An amniocentesis is therefore required to establish the diagnosis with certainty. (For screening see p. 76)
Respiratory	Pulmonary hypoplasia (e.g. following very early preterm rupture of the membranes or Potter syndrome)	Ultrasound scan
Skeletal	Thanatophoric dysplasia, achondrogenesis, osteogenesis imperfecta type II	Ultrasound scan
Multiple Abnormalities	• Cystic hygroma (particularly if associated with aneuploidy) • VATER association – this refers to a condition in which there are vertebral, anal, tracheal or oesophageal and renal lesions. (Also extended to VACTERL by adding cardiac and limb abnormalities.)	Ultrasound scan

SECTION 4

Labour and delivery problems

Antepartum haemorrhage

A 30 year old para 1+0 with a previous spontaneous vaginal delivery and appropriately grown fetus is admitted at term with fresh vaginal bleeding and abdominal pain. On examination she is distressed with pain, pale, her pulse is 100 b.p.m., blood pressure 110/80 mmHg and she has a tender uterus contracting 3:10 min. Although she had tried to clean herself as much as possible, while waiting for the ambulance to transfer her to the maternity unit, you notice that she has blood stains on her feet between her toes.

What is the most likely diagnosis?

The most likely diagnosis is placental abruption. Placental abruption is, by definition, premature separation of the normally implanted placenta from the uterine wall, resulting in haemorrhage prior to delivery of the fetus. It is a major cause of maternal mortality. The cause of placental abruption is usually unknown but abnormal placentation is likely. Risk factors include sudden uterine decompression, external trauma, uterine anomaly, increased maternal age, smoking and an unexplained elevation of maternal serum alphafetoprotein in the second trimester. However, most commonly no cause is found. Bleeding occurs into the decidua basalis of the placenta, which, due to the hydrostatic pressure and development of decidual haematoma, leads to separation of the adjacent placenta. As the uterus is still distended with the pregnancy, it is unable to contract down on the uterine vessels in the placental site, which is the normal haemostatic mechanism to prevent haemorrhage after delivery. The expanding haematoma will dissect between the fetal membranes, leading to vaginal bleeding. However, the bleeding can on occasion be in whole or in part concealed if the haematoma has not reached the margin of the placenta and the cervix, so that the revealed blood loss per se is not an accurate guide to the degree of haemorrhage. The haematoma may also result in bleeding into the amniotic cavity, resulting in blood-stained amniotic fluid when the membranes rupture. In addition, bleeding and haematoma can occur in the myometrium, resulting in the so-called 'Couvelaire uterus', which is associated with sustained uterine contractions resulting in labour and fetal compromise, and also with uterine atony postpartum, which may be a cause of severe postpartum haemorrhage.

It is important to differentiate placental abruption from placenta praevia, the other major cause of a haemorrhage in late pregnancy. Bleeding from placenta praevia is due to the separation of a placenta implanted into the lower uterine segment as a result of the lower segment forming or the cervix dilating. This usually presents with small painless bleeds in the early part of the third trimester, but severe bleeding can occur in association with labour. The characteristic clinical presentation of this condition is painless and often minor degrees of vaginal bleeding, which settle spontaneously. Major degrees of placenta praevia are incompatible with a vaginal delivery and caesarean section is required. Because the placenta is in the lower uterine segment, malpresentation and unstable lie are common. Ultrasound is usually used to delineate the placental site before conservative management is employed. Formation of the lower uterine segment may result in the placenta 'moving' clear of the cervix proper and thus, in minor degrees of this condition, a conservative approach is satisfactory.

What are the risks to the mother and fetus?

The mother's risks relate to the complications of haemorrhage, whether it be antepartum or postpartum. These include hypovolaemic shock, acute renal failure and DIC. Postpartum haemorrhage is more common, not only due to DIC but also because of an atonic uterus following delivery, which may be associated with the Couvelaire uterus. Rhesus sensitization may also occur as a result of significant fetomaternal haemorrhage and all Rhesus-negative mothers who have an abruption should receive anti-D immunoglobulin. Clearly, the volume of fetomaternal haemorrhage may be large and a Kleihauer test should be employed to determine the volume of the haemorrhage and therefore the dose of anti-D necessary.

The problems for the fetus will include premature delivery, either spontaneous or iatrogenic, fetal anaemia due to fetomaternal haemorrhage and/or blood loss from the placenta. Fetal distress can occur due to fetoplacental vasoconstriction, anaemia and uterine hypertonus. It is noteworthy that many of these infants suffer from IUGR. These factors combine to lead to a dramatic increase in the perinatal mortality rate associated with abruption, and this may be in excess of 30%. Furthermore, surviving infants may have significant problems, such as neurological deficit, when followed up. The survival rate will depend on the severity of the abruption, the gestation, birth weight and the amount of concealed haemorrhage.

How should you assess and manage this situation?

The blood loss should be assessed. While it is useful to monitor the degree of vaginal loss, it must be appreciated, as noted above, that the haemorrhage may be in part or in whole concealed (Fig. 44.1) and that it is critical in abruption to monitor pulse, blood pressure, urine output (requiring a urinary catheter) and often central venous pressure. The woman should also be observed for any evidence of clinical shock and uterine activity. Furthermore, there should be an assessment of whether the uterine size might be increasing due to continued intrauterine blood loss. In addition, blood should be taken for coagulation screen, full blood count and cross-matching of a minimum of 4 units of blood; urea and electrolytes may also be useful. An assessment should be made of the fetal condition with CTG and ultrasound scan to confirm viability. Ultrasound scan may also be useful for excluding placenta praevia, which is an important differential diagnosis but may also be a coincidental finding as it may occur in up to 10% of abruptions. Where the retroplacental clot is large, it may be identified on ultrasound. This is not a reliable diagnostic technique. It is essential that in the management of these cases good venous access is obtained as early as possible: ideally, two large-bore intravenous cannulas should be inserted on presentation to allow rapid resuscitation with blood or plasma expanders. It is noteworthy that dextran should not be used in this situation as it can precipitate an anaphylactoid reaction, which can provoke fetal compromise. It is also useful to involve senior obstetricians, haematologists and anaesthetists in the management of these cases,

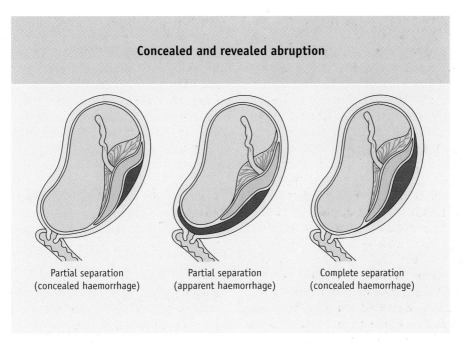

Concealed and revealed abruption

Partial separation
(concealed haemorrhage)

Partial separation
(apparent haemorrhage)

Complete separation
(concealed haemorrhage)

Fig. 44.1   Concealed and revealed abruption.

which can evolve rapidly and have very serious consequences.

One hour later the maternal condition was essentially unchanged from admission. She still has a borderline tachycardia, blood pressure is satisfactory and the uterus continues to contract 3:10 min and remains tender. CTG shows appropriate beat-to-beat variability with no decelerations in response to contractions. The coagulation screen results become available. They show haemoglobin 8.4 g/dl, platelets 105×10^9/l, fibrinogen 2.2 g/l, activated partial thromboplastin time (aPTT) 48 s, prothrombin time 14 s, fibrin degradation products 2.1 mg/ml. Comment on these results and discuss further management.

These results show reduced haemoglobin, reduced fibrinogen and increased fibrin degradation pro-

ducts. It is noteworthy that fibrinogen usually increases dramatically in pregnancy and this value indicates significant consumption of fibrinogen. There is borderline prolongation of the prothrombin time and partial thromboplastin time. Further monitoring is required, as serious haemostatic problems could result with worsening of the aPTT, prothrombin time and a further substantial fall in fibrinogen. The best way to deal with this problem is to effect delivery to prevent further blood loss and coagulation failure. However, blood product therapy, such as infusion of fresh frozen plasma, may be required. Platelet concentrate is normally only required if the platelet count falls to $< 50 \times 10^9$/l, associated with the need for operative delivery or spontaneous bleeding.

As the patient is continuing to contract and therefore appears to be labouring with a significant abruption, she should be taken to theatre for examination, usually without anaesthesia. The theatre should be set for caesarean section, as this might be required if the alternative or coexisting diagnosis of placenta praevia is found or if severe fetal distress occurs (Fig. 44.2).

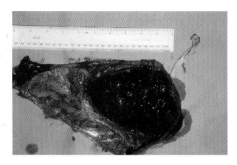

Fig. 44.2 *A large placental abruption showing extensive clot attached to the fetal side of the placenta following delivery by emergency section for severe fetal distress.*

between diagnosis-to-delivery time and the perinatal mortality rate. However, in the absence of fetal distress, labour, which is usually extremely rapid, should be allowed to progress. An oxytocic to augment labour can be used if required. Of particular concern is the high risk of postpartum haemorrhage that these women face following delivery. Should an in utero death have occurred, then vaginal delivery should be anticipated.

On examination the cervix is found to be 5 cm dilated and fully effaced with no placenta palpable. The fetal head is at the level of the ischial spines and is in the left occipitoanterior position. Should you perform amniotomy?

Amniotomy is usually performed in part to enhance labour or, perhaps more importantly, to give a more accurate measure of the fetal condition by allowing a fetal scalp electrode to be attached and also to assess for fresh meconium. If fetal distress occurs, caesarean section should be performed immediately, as there is a close association

You perform an amniotomy and the patient delivers a live male infant less than 1 h later. The infant is healthy with Apgar score of 9 at 5 min. The placenta is rapidly delivered and has approximately 500 ml of clot adhered to about 25% of its surface area. She recovers uneventfully. At her postnatal check the patient asks about the risk of having a similar event in a subsequent pregnancy. What is the risk of such a recurrence?

The risk of recurrent abruption may be as high as 1:8 to 1:12. There is no clear evidence that folate supplements will influence this risk; however, if the patient is a smoker, giving up smoking may substantially reduce the risk of abruption, stillbirth and neonatal death.

Preterm labour

A 34 year old para 1+0 with a previous spontaneous vaginal delivery at 36 weeks gestation of a normally grown infant is admitted to the labour ward at 30 weeks gestation complaining of regular contraction-type pain occurring approximately once every 10 min. Up until this point the pregnancy has been uncomplicated. There is no history of vaginal bleeding and no history of spontaneous rupture of membranes. The midwife who has been attending her from admission indicates to you that she has felt uterine contractions occurring 1–2 in 10 min. She reports that the CTG that she has instituted shows a normal reactive pattern with accelerations occurring in association with each contraction and a normal baseline heart rate of 150 b.p.m. with good variability. You note that she is apyrexial, that the uterine fundal height is compatible with her dates and that the fetus has a longitudinal lie with a cephalic presentation.

What is the likely diagnosis and how would you assess and manage this situation?

The major concern is that this patient is in preterm labour. The diagnosis of labour should be made from documented uterine contractions of at least 1 every 10 min and the presence of ruptured fetal membranes or documented cervical change, an estimated length of the cervix of < 1 cm and/or a cervical dilatation of > 2 cm. The diagnosis of threatened preterm labour may be suspected where there are regular uterine contractions but no evidence of cervical change. It is important, where possible, to make an early diagnosis because of the need for early management of suspected preterm labour. Treatment is often instituted before the diagnosis is absolutely confirmed, as often once labour is well established there is little prospect of intervention.

Thus, in this patient's situation it is important to take an appropriate history, examine the abdomen and perform a speculum and vaginal examination to assess the cervix and look for evidence of cervical dilatation and rupture of membranes and to obtain bacteriological swabs, as infection is a common cause of preterm labour. It is also worth confirming the gestational age and assessing the fetal condition. In this case CTG has already been performed. Clinical signs of possible infection, such as elevated temperature, should be sought.

On speculum and vaginal examination, you find that the cervix is 2 cm dilated and <1 cm long, and bulging forewaters can be felt. There is no evidence of vaginal bleeding and you obtain a high vaginal swab for bacteriological analysis. What further assessment and treatment would you institute at this point?

This patient appears to meet the definition of at least threatened preterm labour, which is most likely to be idiopathic as no precipitant such as preterm premature rupture of the membranes or antepartum haemorrhage has been found, although subclinical infection may be a cause. Where infection is suspected, in addition to a high vaginal swab, midstream specimen of urine, full blood count including white cell count and C-reactive protein may be helpful.

Appropriate treatment at this point must include prophylactic administration of steroids to enhance fetal lung maturity. Evidence from a meta-analysis indicates that the benefits of steroid administration are clear in babies born at the gestation at which this patient presents. The benefits are in terms of a reduction in neonatal death and also morbidity due to respiratory distress syndrome, intraventricular haemorrhage and necrotizing enterocolitis. It should be noted that prelabour preterm rupture of the membranes and suspected or treated infection should not be regarded as contraindications to steroid therapy, as significant benefits may still ensue. The steroids should be given in the form of 12 mg betamethasone intramuscularly on two occasions 24 h apart; however, dexamethasone has also been used for this purpose. There is no evidence that any one regimen is any more effective than another. It is noteworthy that, should the patient be taking enzyme-inducing drugs such as anticonvulsants, the dose of steroids needs to be doubled. Documented benefits from such administration are evidenced between 24 h and 7 days after steroid administration, although there may be some benefit if the fetus is delivered before the initial 24 h has elapsed or beyond the 7 days. Thus, even if delivery is anticipated within 24 h, steroids should still be given.

The next question is whether tocolytic therapy should be used in this situation. Tocolytic therapy is indicated in women presenting with preterm labour under 34 weeks gestation who require transfer to a tertiary centre with appropriate neonatal care facilities or in order to permit steroid administration. The most commonly used tocolytic agent is the beta-mimetic agent, ritodrine, which should be administered intravenously via a controlled infusion device. It has proven efficacy for short-term tocolysis and can delay delivery for more than 24 h; however, this delay is not associated with a significant reduction in respiratory distress syndrome or perinatal death with tocolytic therapy alone. Beta-mimetics have potentially serious maternal side-effects and have been associated with significant morbidity and mortality, thus calling into question the risk: benefit ratio for such therapy. In addition, its effect diminishes after 1–2 days. In view of these concerns, its use should be limited to 48 h with careful control. This drug should not be used in women with cardiac disease, hyperthyroidism, diabetes or hypertension.

Alternative tocolytic therapy includes the use of non-steroidal anti-inflammatory drugs such as indometacin, to inhibit prostaglandin synthase and thereby uterine contractions, and nifedipine, a calcium channel blocker which may also inhibit uterine contractions. These are used in preference to ritodrine in mothers with diabetes.

Thus, with regard to the immediate management of the patient described above, she should receive two doses of betamethasone 12 mg intramuscularly 24 h apart; if there is suspicion that labour is progressing, administration of a tocolytic such as ritodrine, or alternatively indometacin or nifedipine, should be considered to allow steroid administration to take place.

Throughout this time, there should be careful fetal monitoring.

Although subclinical chorioamnionitis may be an important aetiological factor in cases of preterm labour, antibiotics should not be routinely given unless thare is some evidence of infection. A large randomized multicentre trial recently assessed the role of antibiotics in preterm labour. Over 6000 women in spontaneous preterm labour, with intact membranes and without evidence of clinical infection, were randomized to antibiotic therapy or placebo. None of the trial antibiotic regimens was associated with a lower rate of the composite outcome of neonatal death, chronic lung disease or major cerebral abnormality than placebo, but antibiotic prescription was associated with a lower occurrence of maternal infection. Thus antibiotics should not be routinely prescribed for women in spontaneous preterm labour without evidence of clinical infection.

If the patient is not in a facility that can provide tertiary level neonatal care for the infant, transfer to such a unit should be considered, under tocolytic cover, and the paediatricians should be informed of the likely preterm delivery of this infant.

Some 12 h later she is continuing to contract despite tocolytic therapy with ritodrine. Vaginal examination shows the cervix to be 6 cm dilated and fully effaced. The CTG shows a normal baseline heart rate with good beat-to-beat variability and no decelerations. As labour appears to be progressing, what is the optimum mode of delivery for this baby?

In an appropriately grown fetus such as this, at 30 weeks gestation with a cephalic presentation and no evidence of fetal distress, vaginal delivery should be anticipated. Regional analgesia is frequently employed in this situation but there is no need for elective instrumental vaginal delivery except for the usual obstetric indications. An experienced paediatrician should be in attendance for resuscitation at the time of delivery.

Slow progress in labour

A 29 year old primigravid patient is admitted to the labour ward at 01.00 hours. She is at term, having had an uncomplicated pregnancy, and gives a history of show and regular painful contraction-like pain occurring 3:10 min. Just as she was admitted, spontaneous rupture of membranes occurred. On abdominal examination she is found to have a uterine fundal height compatible with term; the fetus has a longitudinal lie and cephalic presentation. On vaginal examination the cervix is found to be 4 cm dilated, fully effaced with the vertex at 0^{-2} station. A fetal scalp electrode is applied for continuous CTG monitoring and, at the patient's request, epidural anaesthesia is administered for analgesia.

Some 4 h later, at 05.00 hours, she is re-examined to assess progress in labour. Two- to three-fifths of the head are palpable abdominally. On vaginal examination the cervix is found to be 5–6 cm dilated, fully effaced with the fetal head at 0^{-1} station. The CTG is satisfactory and the epidural analgesia remains effective. A further 2 h later, at 07.00 hours, she is reassessed by the midwife and found to be 6 cm dilated but otherwise the findings have not changed from the previous assessment. The CTG remained satisfactory.

You are asked to make an assessment of the situation. What do you consider to be the differential diagnosis for her slow progress in labour and how would you manage this?

Slow progress in labour in a primigravida with a longitudinal lie and cephalic presentation is usually due to one of three causes: inefficient uterine contractility, occipitoposterior position of the fetal head, or cephalopelvic disproportion. Clearly unusual situations, such as hydrocephalus, brow presentation and an undiagnosed shoulder presentation, should be excluded.

Inefficient uterine contractility is common in primigravidae. While uterine contractions in this situation may sometimes appear infrequent and of poor strength, it is notoriously difficult to assess the strength of uterine contractions by abdominal palpation. The most reliable evidence of efficient uterine contractility is progressive cervical dilatation, which can be assessed on vaginal examination. The remedy for inefficient uterine contractility is augmentation of labour by oxytocin following amniotomy, if spontaneous rupture of membranes or artificial rupture of membranes has not previously occurred or been performed. The dose of oxytocin should be titrated against contraction frequency. Reassessment within 1–2 h of commencement of oxytocin will determine whether slow progress in labour has been corrected. Care must be taken during the infusion to ensure that uterine hyperstimulation leading to fetal distress does not occur; the infusion is usually controlled by means of an infusion pump. The normal rate of cervical dilatation in a primigravida is approximately 1 cm/h.

Occipitoposterior position of the fetal head presents a larger diameter to the maternal pelvis than the occipitoanterior vertex presentation, which is the more common position for the fetal head in labour. Occipitoposterior position is associated with the fetal head being deflexed and the diameter presented to the maternal pelvis is the occipitofrontal diameter, rather than the suboccipitobregmatic diameter seen in a well-flexed head with the vertex presenting. The difference in diameter is approximately 1 cm. The reason why occipitoposterior position occurs may be related to the head failing to flex adequately, which in turn may be due to inefficient uterine contractility. In early labour there is compaction and flexion of the fetus; in the presence of inefficient uterine activity this process may fail and thus the head remains deflexed. The shape of the pelvic floor is such that the first part of the fetal head to strike the pelvic floor will rotate anteriorly. With a well-flexed fetal head the first part to encounter the pelvic floor will be close to the occiput, and thus the occiput will rotate anteriorly. With a deflexed fetal head the part of the head that will strike the pelvic floor first will be close to the anterior fontanelle, and thus the anterior part of the head tends to rotate anteriorly or may arrest in a transverse position. Diagnosis of occipitoposterior or occipitotrans-verse positions can be easily made on vaginal examination, by palpation of the fontanelle and suture lines. In the first stage of labour, the combination of slow progress in terms of cervical dilatation coupled with the finding of occipitoposterior or occipitotransverse position should in the first instance be treated with augmentation by oxytocin infusion, as noted above. Progress should be evident within 1–2 h of appropriate administration of oxytocin. On occasion the head may fail to rotate anteriorly and descend and caesarean section may be required. On other occasions the cervix may progress to full dilatation with the head in an occipitoposterior or occipitotransverse position at or below the level of the ischial spines, and in this situation rotational delivery by ventouse or Kielland's forceps may be possible.

Cephalopelvic disproportion is essentially a diagnosis of exclusion. To make this diagnosis inefficient uterine contractility and occipitoposterior position of the fetal head should be excluded by examination and augmentation of labour by oxytocin. If augmentation has occurred and there is still failure of progress in the first stage of labour, the delivery should be by caesarean section with a presumptive diagnosis of cephalopelvic disproportion, provided that occipitoposterior or occipitotransverse position has been excluded. Where occipitotransverse or occipitoposterior position occurs, this does not necessarily indicate cephalopelvic disproportion because, if the fetal head had been well flexed with the vertex presenting with the smaller diameter in an optimal position, i.e. occipitoanterior, delivery might have been possible. Nonetheless caesarean section will still be required if progress fails to occur. Other presumptive evidence for the diagnosis of cephalopelvic disproportion would be excessive moulding, i.e. overlapping of the fetal skull bones.

Thus, in a situation of a primigravida with a cephalic presentation making slow progress, the diagnosis lies between inefficient uterine contractility, occipitoposterior position and cephalopelvic disproportion. Occipitoposterior position can be diagnosed on vaginal examination and should be treated with oxytocin infusion. Failure to progress beyond this will precipitate delivery by caesarean section. Inefficient uterine contractility should be treated with intravenous oxytocin infusion, and a failure to progress in this situation in the absence of occipitoposterior or occipitotransverse position is compatible with cephalopelvic disproportion. When labour is augmented with oxytocin the fetal heart rate should be carefully and continuously monitored for any evidence of fetal distress.

You examine the patient and find that the presenting part is the vertex in the left occipitoanterior position; the cervix is 6 cm dilated and the vertex is 1 cm above the ischial spines. You prescribe intravenous oxytocin, 10 units in 500 ml dextrose in escalating doses by infusion pump, and plan to assess her in 2 h. Two hours later you assess her. She has uterine contractions 3:10 min and two- to three-fifths of the fetal head are palpable abdominally. The cervix is 6–7 cm dilated, the vertex remains at 0^{-1} station and irreducible overlap of the fetal skull bones is present on two of the three palpable suture lines. What is the diagnosis and how should you deliver the patient?

Your presumptive diagnosis is cephalopelvic disproportion as occipitoposterior position has been excluded and she has received an appropriate dose of oxytocin to augment labour. In addition, there is excessive moulding of the fetal head and delivery should be by emergency caesarean section.

What advice should you give for future pregnancies?

In future pregnancies progressing to term there will be a high likelihood of cephalopelvic disproportion recurring and most obstetricians would offer the woman elective caesarean section at 39 weeks gestation. Where possible, it is best to delay elective section until 39 weeks to minimize the risk of respiratory problems for the baby.

Induction of labour

Your patient is a 38 year old primigravida. She conceived following in vitro fertilization after 5 years of unexplained primary infertility. Throughout the pregnancy she has been very anxious with regard to the outcome. She feels it is likely to be her only pregnancy. The pregnancy has been essentially uncomplicated until the latter part of the third trimester, when her uterus has been noted to be small for dates from 34 weeks gestation. Ultrasound scan has estimated the fetal weight to be around the 10th centile for gestation and there has been no fall-off in growth between 34 weeks and 40 weeks, her current gestation, on fortnightly scans. In view of the circumstances, she was monitored regularly for fetal well-being by way of biophysical profiles and these have invariably been satisfactory. In addition, umbilical artery Doppler flow velocity waveforms are normal. The only other feature of note is the presence of hypertension, blood pressure being 140/98 mmHg, confirmed at the last day care visit, when she had fetal monitoring performed. Biochemistry is normal and there is no proteinuria. Booking blood pressure was 120/80 mmHg. She and her partner request induction of labour the following day, when she will be 40+2 weeks gestation. The dates are certain, as conception was by in vitro fertilization and confirmed by subsequent ultrasound scans.

Is induction of labour warranted in this patient?

Perhaps the most important decision with regard to the process of induction of labour is not the choice or method but whether or not the induction is warranted. The obstetrician must be clear with regard to the balance of risks that exist between continuing with the pregnancy and interrupting it. In this case, there would appear good grounds to proceed to induction of labour in view of several features.

The fetus is small for dates and, although there is no evidence of fetal compromise, this has created significant anxiety and need for regular fetal assessment, which, in addition to the pregnancy being conceived by in vitro fertilization after prolonged primary infertility, are significant causes of maternal anxiety and obstetric concern. In addition, she now has a degree of hypertension. This is relatively modest. There is no evidence of pre-eclampsia. However, such hypertension is a cause for concern in this patient as it may be associated with developing pregnancy-induced hypertension. Thus, there is sufficient cause to warrant induction of labour in this case.

What further assessment would you make before making a decision with regard to induction?

It is important to assess fetal well-being if this has not already been confirmed. Abdominal palpation should be performed to confirm that the presentation is cephalic, the lie longitudinal and that the head is entering the pelvis. Engagement should also be determined. The most important component of the assessment, however, is that of the cervical score, which is useful in providing a degree of objectivity to the assessment. These scores give a prediction of the type of labour and outcome to be expected. If the cervix is ripe, a relatively short and easy labour with little additional stress to the fetus may be anticipated, whereas in the case of a very unripe cervix, the converse will apply. The cervical scoring system is usually used as shown in Table 47.1. If the score is < 7, cervical ripening is required.

Where the cervix is ripe, it would be anticipated that induction would be straightforward.

Where the cervix is very unripe, one option is to defer delivery in anticipation of a spontaneous increase in ripening; however, this is essentially a temporary measure, as the factors that precipitate the need for intervention are more likely to worsen than recede with time, and this is likely to be the case with the present patient. The next alternative is to proceed to caesarean section, which minimizes the stress for the fetus but increases the risk of morbidity to the mother. The third possible option is to achieve cervical ripening pharmacologically as a prelude to induction of labour.

On examination, the fetus has a longitudinal lie with a cephalic presentation and three-fifths of the head are palpable within the abdomen. On vaginal examination, the cervix is found to be <1 cm dilated, 2-4 cm long, medium consistency, midanterior position and the station of the fetal head is 0^{-3}. What is the cervical score and what management option would you take?

The cervical score is 3, based on the scoring system in Table 47.1. A score of 0–3 might be regarded as unripe, 4–7 intermediate and 8–11 ripe; thus, the cervix is not ripe and in its present condition is not favourable for induction. The options available are noted above, i.e. deferred delivery, perform caesarean section or achieve cervical ripening. In this patient's case, in the absence of any evidence of fetal compromise, there would

Table 47.1 The modified Bishop scoring system for cervical assessment

	Score			
	0	1	2	3
Cervical dilatation (cm)	<1	1–2	3–4	>4
Length of cervix (cm)	>4	2–4	1–2	<1
Station of presenting part (cm)	Spines–3	Spines–2	Spines–1	–
Consistency	Firm	Average	Soft	–
Position	Posterior	Mid/anterior		–

be no compelling reason to proceed immediately to caesarean section and in the first instance an attempt at cervical ripening should be made. If this is successful, then a straightforward induction may occur, avoiding the need for caesarean section.

How would you perform cervical ripening in this patient?

A variety of methods exist for cervical ripening. These include physical techniques, such as the insertion of Foley catheters, and pharmacological techniques, usually utilising prostaglandins. The most commonly administered prostaglandin for cervical ripening is prostaglandin E_2 (PGE_2), which may be administered in a variety of preparations. The ideal preparation for cervical ripening should produce a satisfactory effect on the cervix while avoiding stimulation of myometrial activity. Clearly the overall goal of the intervention process is to induce labour and, while myometrial activity may not, at first sight, seem to be of serious concern, such activity in the absence of a compliant cervix will result in increased stress to mother and fetus, with a higher incidence of problems such as fetal distress and operative delivery. Vaginal administration of prostaglandins in gel or vaginal tablet form is optimal for maximum efficacy with minimal side-effects. Extra-amniotic and endocervical applications of prostaglandins have also been used. While the extra-amniotic route of prostaglandin administration via a Foley catheter is known to be highly effective, it is invasive, with a small risk of infection and the possibility of bleeding into the choriodecidual space, which could lead to uterine hypertonus due to rapid uptake of prostaglandins. The invasiveness of the technique may be disagreeable for the patient. Endocervical application of PGE_2 has also been used but does require a degree of skill to effect placement of the gel accurately in the cervical canal, avoiding placement into the extra-amniotic space and also leakage from the external os into the vagina.

In this patient, it would be reasonable to effect cervical ripening with vaginal administration of PGE_2. A suitable regimen to follow with this patient would be to admit her at around 1600 hours the following day, confirm fetal well-being and check the findings on abdominal palpation. Thereafter, the cervical score should be reassessed and, if less than 7, 2 mg PGE_2 gel should be inserted vaginally. She should be left overnight to allow maximal ripening and reassessed at 0900 hours the following morning. If the cervix has ripened, formal induction of labour can occur at this point. If insufficient ripening has occurred, further PGE_2 gel in a dose of 1 or 2 mg, depending on the cervical state, can be given. Fetal monitoring by way of CTG should be performed after PGE_2 administration and if uterine contractility develops.

Following administration of the PGE_2 vaginal gel, she has some irregular uterine tightenings. The CTG confirms fetal well-being; she sleeps overnight without any need for analgesia. The following morning you reassess her at 0900 hours. She has irregular uterine activity and the CTG remains reactive. On vaginal examination you find that the cervix is now fully effaced, i.e. <1 cm long, 3–4 cm dilated, soft in consistency, central in position and the station of the fetal head at 0^{-2}. What is the cervical score and how would you perform induction?

The cervical score is 9, thus the cervix is now ripe. The induction may be best effected by amniotomy, followed by intravenous oxytocin if regular contractions do not develop following the amniotomy. Continuous CTG monitoring is essential during induction of labour.

You perform artificial rupture of the membranes (Fig. 47.1), the amniotic fluid is clear with no evidence of meconium staining, and you attach a fetal scalp electrode in order to monitor the fetus carefully during labour. One hour later you review her as she is requesting

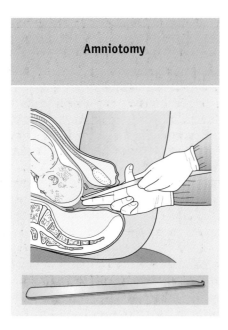

Amniotomy

Fig. 47.1   *Artificial rupture of the membranes.*

analgesia. She is contracting regularly 3:10 min and after discussion she decides to have epidural anaesthesia. This is established by the anaesthetist and you review her again 2 h later to assess progress. Abdominal examination is unchanged from before, the CTG shows no abnormality and on vaginal examination the cervix is fully effaced, 7 cm dilated, well applied to the fetal head, soft in consistency and the fetal head is at 0^{-2} station. Is there need for augmentation with oxytocin at this point?

The patient is now in established labour and making good progress for a primigravida following induction. A satisfactory rate of progress, once labour is established, can be considered to be around 1 cm/h. Thus, this patient does not need augmentation with oxytocin at the present time.

You are next asked to see her some 4 h later when she has been in the second

stage of labour for 55 min, with active pushing for the last 30 min. You have been called because the midwife is concerned about frequent variable decelerations associated with meconium-stained liquor. The midwife reports that when she diagnosed full dilatation the vertex was 1 cm below the ischial spines. You review the CTG and see that occasional variable decelerations were present over the last 2 h but over the last 15 min these have occurred with minimal respite, and the baseline fetal heart rate has increased to 170–180 beats/min. The meconium in the liquor appears fresh. The medical student on the labour ward asks you if you would perform a fetal blood sample. Would a fetal blood sample be merited and what action would you take?

Persistent variable decelerations, often associated with umbilical cord compression, and fetal tachycardia are CTG patterns that are associated with fetal compromise, particularly in a fetus that is already at risk, such as those who are small for dates or growth restricted. The presence of fresh meconium can also indicate fetal distress. Thus, there is sufficient information available to warrant a presumptive diagnosis of fetal distress. As she is in the second stage of labour with the vertex below the ischial spines, delivery is likely to be be possible by forceps or ventouse. There is unlikely to be any benefit in performing a fetal blood sample. Where there is real suspicion of fetal distress in the second stage of labour, delivery should be expedited.

You perform vaginal examination and find that the fetal head is in the occipitoanterior position 2 cm below the ischial spines. There is no moulding but significant caput is present. You confirm that the cervix is fully dilated. You decide to perform a forceps delivery; what

measures should you take prior to carrying out such an assisted vaginal delivery?

You should ensure that adequate analgesia is in place, the epidural should be topped up, if not fully effective. If there is insufficient time for this, a pudendal nerve block can be performed. The bladder should be emptied using a urinary catheter to avoid bladder injury and facilitate delivery. You should confirm full dilatation, the station and position of the head.

In the course of the forceps delivery, once descent of the head is evident and the perineum stretching, an episiotomy should be performed. As frequent variable decelerations may be associated with cord compression or with a cord tight around the neck, it is useful immediately the head is delivered to check for nuchal cord and divide it or pull it over the baby's head prior to delivering the body. In this case, forceps delivery is straightforward and is effected over two contractions. Nuchal cord is noted. This is tight and needs to be divided in situ before completing delivery of the baby. The baby is delivered with Apgar scores of 4 at 1 min and 9 at 5 min. The paediatrician assesses the baby following delivery and finds, on laryngoscopy, that there is no evidence of meconium below the level of the vocal cords (meconium aspiration can cause respiratory problems in the baby, which can be severe). The baby's condition appears stable and satisfactory and he remains in the labour ward with his parents. You deliver the placenta by controlled cord traction and suture the episiotomy.

Post-dates pregnancy

A 42 year old primigravida is seen in the antenatal clinic at 40 weeks gestation. She has been investigated in her late 20s for primary infertility and told that, because her fallopian tubes did not seem to be patent, it was unlikely that she would ever conceive spontaneously. Having slowly come to terms with her infertility, it had been with astonishment, and very great joy, that she at last found herself pregnant. The pregnancy has passed uneventfully and now, at 40 weeks, she shows you her extensive birth plan, adamant that she wishes to await labour naturally, no matter how much further the pregnancy carries on.

What information would you wish to know before counselling this patient?

Most importantly, it is essential to ensure that her dates are correct. Establishing gestational age by ultrasound scan is relatively accurate up to 18–20 weeks, as there is little variation in growth between different fetuses. After this time, accuracy is reduced and by the third trimester precise dating is impossible. In this case the patient had an ultrasound scan at 10 weeks gestation, and this correlated well with her own estimated gestation from the last menstrual period.

Next, it is important to ensure that there are no other complications to put the pregnancy at a higher risk. Is there any evidence of pre-eclampsia (check blood pressure and urinalysis), IUGR (check abdominal palpation and if in doubt organize an ultrasound scan) or fetal compromise (are there plenty of movements)? Are the lie and presentation normal?

How would you advise this couple?

It would be considered appropriate by many obstetricians to offer induction of labour at between 7 and 11 days after the due date, although up to 14 days may be quite acceptable. After this time the fetus is said to be 'post-term', and between 4 and 14% of women will reach this stage of pregnancy. Perinatal mortality is increased, the main cause of death being classified as 'unexplained'. Perinatal morbidity is also increased (as indicated by an increase in the incidence of neonatal seizures, a strong marker for neonatal encephalopathy). If a woman chooses to continue the pregnancy beyond 42 weeks then regular fetal monitoring, such as twice- to thrice-weekly biophysical profiles could be instituted because of the risk to the fetus.

Although induction of labour at or before 40 weeks is associated with an increased chance of requiring forceps or a caesarean section over spontaneous labour, this is not true at 41–42 weeks. Spontaneous labour after 42 weeks is again associated with an increased chance of caesarean section and forceps over earlier induction of labour (usually for reasons of fetal compromise). In general, therefore, there is evidence that induction of labour between 41 and 42 weeks is in both the maternal and fetal interest, reducing intervention and perinatal death.

In this particular case, there is even more reason to advise intervention as the risk of perinatal mortality is likely to be further increased because of advanced maternal age. She is very unlikely to have the chance to have any other children, and it is therefore even more important to ensure that she has a good outcome on this occasion.

They accept your advice willingly, and a date for induction is set for 10 days

hence. Before they leave, you mention a 'membrane sweep' to them. What is this and is it beneficial?

This involves a vaginal examination. A finger is slipped through the cervical os and the membranes separated (i.e. 'swept away') from the uterine wall, increasing the local release of prostaglandins. Prostaglandins are thought to be mediators in the initiation of labour. Sweeping the membranes at or after 40 weeks doubles the incidence of spontaneous labour over controls. The risk of infection is considered to be minimal. The procedure is uncomfortable.

The night after the membrane sweep she is admitted in spontaneous labour. In the meantime, you are approached by the hospital administrator, concerned at the number of labour inductions. He wonders if this will lead to complaints from parents at not being allowed to labour naturally. What advice would you offer?

There is evidence that dissatisfaction with labour is strongly associated with operative delivery and is not associated with induction of labour.

Preterm rupture of membranes

A 19 year old para 0+1 (previous suction termination of pregnancy at 12 weeks gestation) presents at 25 weeks in her second pregnancy. She had been watching television when all of a sudden she felt a leakage of water on her trousers. She was concerned, but went to bed at her usual time and was woken twice during the night with further gushes of fluid. She has not had pain but is now, the next morning, worried that something might be wrong.

Are her worries justified and why?

It is possible that she has been having episodes of stress incontinence, but on further questioning she says that she had emptied her bladder just half an hour before the first leak, and that there has been more fluid coming away than she would have expected, particularly as she hasn't been drinking much liquid. Furthermore, she did not think it smelled of urine. The most likely diagnosis is of preterm prelabour rupture of membranes and her concerns are therefore definitely justified.

Most mothers with preterm rupture of membranes will establish in spontaneous labour within the subsequent 1–2 weeks and the neonatal mortality for a baby born at 25 weeks gestation is likely to be in excess of 500/1000. In addition, there is a significant risk of perinatal morbidity and the possibity of long-term physical or mental inpairment. There is also a small risk of ascending infection leading to chorioamnionitis, which carries potentially serious risks for both mother and baby.

What would you look for on examination and what investigations would you perform?

Review the past history (membrane rupture is more common with twins or with polyhydramnios). If there is chorioamnionitis, the temperature may be raised and the uterus tender. Check that the fetal heartbeat is present (fetal tachycardia may indicate infection) and try to ascertain the lie and presentation (which may be very difficult at 25 weeks). Ask if she is wearing a sanitary pad and ask if you might look at it. If soaked with fluid, membrane rupture is likely.

Prepare to carry out an aseptic speculum examination. Inspect the introitus, looking for umbilical cord (cord prolapse) or fluid leakage (do not confuse your antiseptic solution for liquor). Ask her to cough (looking for urinary leakage per urethra with stress incontinence or liquor leakage per vaginam with ruptured membranes).

If liquor is definitely seen, many clinicians would not proceed to any vaginal examination at all because of the risk of introducing infection. Others consider a speculum examination useful to visualize the cervix, exclude cord prolapse and allow a high vaginal swab to be sent to bacteriology (infection is associated with preterm membrane rupture, particularly with the group B haemolytic streptococcus, *Escherichia coli* and *Bacteroides* spp). If liquor is not seen at the introitus, perform a speculum examination with a good light. A pool of liquor may be seen in the posterior fornix, or liquor may be seen coming from the os with further coughing.

Send the high vaginal swab for immediate Gram staining, and send bloods for a white cell count and C-reactive protein (elevated in infection). Arrange an ultrasound scan to confirm presentation, measure the liquor volume (reduced with membrane rupture) and check baseline fetal growth measurements.

Clinical examination confirms membrane rupture. There is no clinical evidence of infection and the baby is cephalic on ultrasound scan, with growth measurements on the 50th centile. What would be your further management plan?

Management involves striking a balance between delivering too soon (with its risks of fetal morbidity and mortality) or not delivering (and developing chorioamnionitis). At 25 weeks gestation, the risks of delivery almost certainly far outweigh conservative management and it would be preferable to monitor the pregnancy closely in the hope of allowing it to proceed as far as possible, ideally well into the third trimester:

- Avoid vaginal examinations, unless there is very good reason to believe that the mother is in labour.
- Give steroids (dexamethasone or betamethasone 24 mg i.m. over 24 h) in case of preterm delivery. This stimulates surfactant production from the type II pneumocytes in the alveoli.
- Give a course of broad-spectrum antibiotics irrespective of bacteriological findings: there is evidence that this prolongs the pregnancy. Also treat clinically significant infection based on the sensitivity of vaginal swabs.
- Monitor for infection, e.g. by checking the temperature four times daily and carrying out twice-weekly C-reactive protein measurements. (The white cell count will be artificially elevated after the steroid treatment).
- Monitor the fetus, e.g. daily checks for the presence of the fetal heartbeat, thrice-weekly ultrasound assessment of fetal tone, breathing and movement, and fortnightly scans for growth. From 27–28 weeks, a CTG may be performed. Measuring the amniotic fluid volume is of little practical use.
- Deliver if chorioamnionitis develops, if there is fetal compromise, or if 34–37 weeks gestation is reached. In the presence of chorioamnionitis or fetal compromise, it is appropriate to perform a caesarean section unless labour is well advanced.

How would you counsel the mother?

The seriousness of the situation should be explained honestly to the parents and the management plan outlined as above (the outcome becomes more guarded the earlier membrane rupture occurs on account of pulmonary hypoplasia and skeletal deformities). Ideally the parents should be offered the opportunity to meet the paediatrician and to visit the neonatal intensive care unit to help understand what might be involved.

She has no children to look after at home and may therefore be willing to stay in hospital for the remainder of her pregnancy. Some clinicians, however, would consider outpatient monitoring after a period of inpatient assessment. Sexual intercourse should be avoided as there is a risk of introducing infection. It would also be reasonable to advise her that this membrane rupture is unlikely to be related to her previous termination of pregnancy (to alleviate potential feelings of guilt).

Intrauterine death

A 42 year old para 1+2 presents at 32 weeks gestation having felt non-specifically unwell for 24 h. She has not felt the baby kicking over this time, and when the midwife tries to perform a CTG she is unable to hear a heartbeat. You are called to see her.

What is your initial management?

It is highly likely that the baby has died in utero. It is clearly essential to diagnose this with certainty and an ultrasound scan is required by somebody with sufficient experience to give definite confirmation of the diagnosis. Assuming that there is no fetal heart activity, the ultrasonographer should briefly look for any obvious reason why the baby might have died, particularly for evidence of IUGR, hydrops fetalis, or structural abnormality. While the placenta should also be checked to exclude abruption, it is important to note that the majority of placental abruptions are not evident on scan.

The bad news should then be broken to the parents, and they should be allowed to share some time together to come to terms with their loss.

The parents want to know what should happen next. What would you say?

The baby clearly needs to be delivered. In the absence of chorioamnionitis, deteriorating coagu-lopathy or placenta praevia, it is likely to be safer to deliver the baby vaginally rather than by cae-sarean section. This avoids unnecessary surgery and its attendant complications. Explain that labour will need to be induced and the ways that this might be possible (see below).

Next, explain that it is important to try to establish why the baby has died. She had been feeling unwell over the preceding 48 h. This could be coincidental but she may have developed pre-eclampsia (check blood pressure and urine) or may have had an infection (send a mid-stream urine specimen, and serum for toxoplasmosis, rubella, cytomegalovirus and Parvovirus B19 virus). Examine for any clinical evidence of abruption, in particular uterine tenderness. Also send blood for full blood count (may be anaemic following abruption), Kleihauer–Betke stain (? feto-maternal transfusion), and HbA_{1c} and random glucose to exclude impaired glucose tolerance. It is also worth checking lupus anticoagulant, anticar-diolipin antibodies and a thrombophilia screen, as these are also associated with impaired fetal outcome (see p. 128).

How would you manage induction and delivery?

Labour is probably most effectively induced in this situation by giving the antiprogestogen mifepristone, followed 48 h later by vaginal and oral prostaglandins, or prostaglandin analogues (e.g. misoprostol). Although many couples are happy to take the mifepristone and often even go home for the 48 h wait, others are keen to stay in for immediate prostaglandin induction. This is also a reasonable course of action and the parents should be allowed to make their own decisions.

The loss of a baby at any stage in pregnancy is extremely traumatic, but particularly at such an advanced gestation. Emotions will be running high and may spill over into anger. Listening is often more useful than speaking. At this stage, the couple may wish to talk about how to tell their friends, relatives and existing children.

As labour progresses it is important not to rupture the membranes until as late as possible, as the risk of ascending chorioamnionitis is higher than with live birth. The mother should be offered appropriate analgesia, including an epidural if required.

What arrangements would you wish to make after the baby has been born?

The parents should be offered the chance to hold their baby and to spend some time together. This is often very difficult for most parents, but important and rarely regretted. It is still important to offer the parents this option even if the baby is malformed, as imagination is usually worse than reality. They should be offered religious support and the chance to take photographs, handprints or a lock of hair.

The parents will need to register the baby and may wish to give him or her a name. Funeral arrangements will need to made, either through the hospital or privately, according to the parents wishes and customs. A postmortem examination often gives extremely useful information, which may be important for subsequent pregnancies and should be encouraged.

Subsequent antenatal clinic appointments should be cancelled and arrangements made for follow-up, ideally by the patient's consultant, to discuss any results and their implications for the future. The parents should be given the contact numbers for any local support group, e.g. SANDS (Stillbirth and Neonatal Death Society). They may also wish to discuss contraception at this stage.

Breech presentation

A 34 year old para 1+1, who is a solicitor, attends your antenatal clinic at 36 weeks gestation. In her first pregnancy she had an uneventful spontaneous vaginal delivery at term and 2 years later had an early miscarriage. She has, so far, had a straightforward time with this pregnancy but has been diagnosed as having a breech presentation on ultrasound scan. In view of the positive memories she has of her last delivery, she asks you about 'going for a natural birth' again.

How would you assess the situation?

Examine the mother and the scan report. Are there any predisposing factors to account for the mal-presentation (e.g. placenta praevia, polyhydramnios, oligohydramnios or fibroids)? What is the baby's weight and on which centile does this weight lie? Has the baby been scanned for fetal abnormality (neural tube defects are very slightly more common with breech presentation)? Is this a frank breech (baby's feet behind its ears), flexed breech (as if the baby was kneeling) or footling (one or both feet hanging down)?

What are this patient's options and what are the advantages and disadvantages of each?

It is reasonable to begin by saying that this is a controversial area. Explain that you will discuss the pros and cons of the different available options and will be guided by her and her partner's decision.

An attempt at external cephalic version is highly recommended. This involves rotating the fetus round to cephalic presentation by abdominal palpation and carries success rates of probably greater than 50% in parous women if performed after 37 weeks gestation. Only a very small percentage revert to breech again. It is less likely to be successful if the breech is engaged in the pelvis, there is oligohydramnios or if the mother is nulliparous. It is easier in the non-frank breech with a free presenting part and posterior placenta.

The version is carried out using intermittent ultrasound guidance, and complications are very rare. Abruptio placentae or fetomaternal haemorrhage have been reported, however, and it is important to have facilities for delivering the baby by caesarean section if problems arise. Rhesus immunoglobulin should be given to all rhesus-negative mothers after the procedure. In this case the patient does not have any known contraindications (IUGR, pre-eclampsia, established rhesus disease or a history of antepartum haemorrhage).

If the version is unsuccessful, the couple's options are to consider either elective caesarean section or planned vaginal delivery; however, there is now good evidence that elective caesarean section is safer for the baby than planned vaginal delivery. The Term Breech Trial Collaborative Group recently reported a study involving 2088 women with a breech presentation at term. Women with large babies or with other contraindications to a vaginal breech delivery were not included. The women were randomly assigned to have either a caesarean section or a planned vaginal breech delivery. They found that around 43% of the women with a planned vaginal breech delivery were delivered by caesarean section, mostly because of complications in labour. There were a lower number of baby deaths and serious problems in those delivered by caesarean section, with 5% of babies born vaginally having such problems compared with only 1.6% of those delivered by caesarean section. It was calculated that, for every additional 14 caesareans carried out, one baby death or serious problem would be avoided. There was no overall difference in complications for the mother in the first 6 weeks after delivery between the two groups.

If vaginal breech delivery is to be undertaken, favourable features include a frank breech, those with an estimated fetal weight between 2500 and 3800 g, and with no evidence of fetal abnormality or compromise. There is, however, a small chance of serious fetal problems complicating the delivery, including intracranial injury, damage to internal organs, spinal cord transection, umbilical cord prolapse and hypoxia following obstruction of the aftercoming head. Umbilical cord prolapse is also more likely in a flexed or footling breech, and obstruction probably more common in larger babies. Obstruction of the aftercoming head may occur too late for useful intervention by either caesarean section or potentially harmful symphysiotomy. If a vaginal breech delivery is planned, it is prudent to use continuous CTG monitoring and resort to caesarean section if obstruction is suspected. Oxytocin should be used only with great caution, if at all.

With elective caesarean section the fetus is usually delivered without difficulty, but there is a small increased risk of maternal morbidity and mortality from venous thromboembolic disease, infection, haemorrhage, operative complications and anaesthetic complications. This morbidity is substantially reduced with thromboprophylaxis, pro-phylactic antibiotics and regional anaesthesia. Although these risks are small, there are also fetal and maternal implications for subsequent pregnancies with the possibility of scar dehiscence. Again, however, this risk is relatively small ($\sim 1\%$).

After considering these three options carefully, she decides to opt for an external cephalic version. Unfortunately this is unsucessful and she opts for caesarean section. What advice would you give for between now and the time the baby delivers?

It is important for her to attend if she is at all suspicious of labour starting, and particularly if her membranes rupture.

It is also important to document the plan for caesarean section in case labour begins before the expected time, and worth saying that, if she presents in advanced labour, it may be too late for a caesarean section. Vaginal delivery in those patients arriving in advanced labour is usually uneventful.

She establishes in labour spontaneously a week later, presenting on the labour ward in the second stage with the desire to push. On the last assessment the breech is frank and the baby's estimated weight 2.9 kg. How would you manage this stage of the labour?

It is probably too late to establish a regional anaesthetic block. With continuous fetal heart monitoring, allow pushing to commence and, as the breech advances, place the mother in lithotomy position. With asepsis, infiltrate the perineum with lignocaine. When the perineum becomes distended, perform an episiotomy. It is then very important to allow the breech to be born by maternal expulsive effort: this allows the head to flex and therefore engage more easily in the pelvis (Fig. 51.1). If the legs are flexed, they should be freed as the breech passes over the introitus. When the trunk is

155

delivered, use a warm moist cloth to hold the baby's pelvis and legs and deliver the anterior arm by flexion over the chest. The posterior shoulder is delivered by rotating the back anteriorly and flexing the other arm.

Allow the baby to hang downwards so that the head will flex and engage into the pelvis. The preferred method for then delivering the head is with forceps (Fig. 51.1H), but the Mauriceau–Smellie–Veit technique may also be used (Fig. 51.1G).

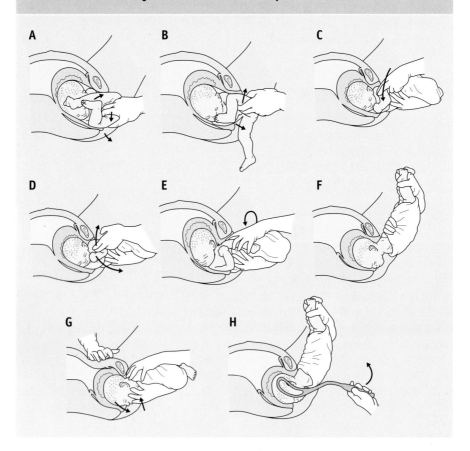

Breech delivery

A flexion of left knee with a frank breech presenting left sacrotransverse
B flexion of left knee
C flexion of the left arm for
D delivery under the symphisis pubis
E rotation of the back anteriorly allows delivery of the posterior shoulder
F lifting the body after allowing the breech to hang
G Mauriceau–Smellie–Veit for head delivery
H alternative delivery of the head with forceps

Fig. 51.1 Breech delivery.

Are there any postnatal considerations?

All babies who have been presenting by the breech should be checked for congenital dislocation of the hip. Those delivered vaginally should also be checked for other possible injuries, including Klumpke paralysis (C8, T1) and the complications mentioned above.

Rupture of membranes prior to labour at term

An 18 year old primigravida is admitted at 38 weeks gestation with a history of having passed a gush of fluid per vaginam. She and her boyfriend had intercourse an hour previously, partly because a friend had advised this as a reliable method of inducing labour. On admission she was undistressed, with a soft non-tender uterus and a fetus in cephalic presentation. The head was four-fifths palpable above the pelvic brim and the CTG was normal.

How would you confirm the diagnosis of membrane rupture?

Although the history is helpful, it is also important to confirm the diagnosis by clinical examination. Liquor may be seen draining from the introitus, and may be further confirmed by the presence of flecks of vernix or meconium. On speculum examination, there is often a pool of fluid sitting in the posterior fornix or seen to be coming from the os when the patient is asked to cough. In the absence of contractions, there is no indication for performing a digital examination, as this risks introducing infection.

Nitrazine sticks have a pH-sensitive orange tip which changes to black when exposed to liquor (amniotic fluid is alkali, maternal urine is acidic).

Unfortunately, as the colour change is dependent only on pH, there may be false results with vaginal discharge, semen (relevant in this case) and blood.

Speculum examination reveals clear liquor draining. If left alone, what is the natural history of events?

Approximately 70% will establish in labour within the subsequent 24 h, and 90% by 48 h. Complications are unusual. Only very rarely does the umbilical cord prolapse (although this is most likely when the head is high, as in this case). The more likely, although still rare (2–3%), complication is of ascending infection which may lead to chorioamnionitis and neonatal infection.

How would you manage this case?

There is some evidence that delaying induction for 2–4 days and allowing labour to establish spontaneously reduces the chance of having to have a casearean section. Evidence from a much larger study however, suggests that this is not the case, and goes on to suggest that induction of labour on admission may be associated with a reduction in chorioamnionitis. There may, in addition, be neonatal benefits and less maternal dissatisfaction with the overall labour process.

Nonetheless, conservative management remains an acceptable option and the choices should be discussed with the parents. Practice varies as to whether the conservatively managed patients should be kept in hospital or allowed home, but in any event a baseline temperature, CTG and palpation should be performed and the mother should be advised to report pains, bleeding, fever, reduced movements or any change in the colour of the liquor.

She opts for conservative management rather than immediate induction. Twelve hours later, she notices that the liquor has turned a greeny/brown colour. How would this affect your management plan?

It is likely that the baby has passed meconium. This has an association with fetal distress and it is therefore important to check a CTG. If this does suggest fetal compromise and the cervix is insufficiently dilated to perform a fetal blood sample, the baby should be delivered at once (i.e. by casearean section). If the CTG is normal, labour should be induced using either prostaglandins if the Bishop score is < 7, or intravenous syntocinon if 7 or more (see p. 143).

Suspected fetal distress in labour

A 40 year old para 3+0 herbalist is admitted at 38 weeks, 2 h after spontaneous rupture of the membranes. She is starting to feel some contractions. All three of her children were born by uncomplicated spontaneous vaginal delivery and, as she is in a relatively low-risk situation, she is keen for delivery to be as natural as possible.

She requests only intermittent fetal heart auscultation rather than continuous CTG. What are CTGs and is her request reasonable?

A cardiotocograph measures fetal heart rate together with the timing of contractions. The routine use of continuous CTG monitoring in low-risk labours may increase the rate of intervention for no demonstrable fetal benefit. It is therefore a very reasonable request, providing the labour is 'low-risk'.

How would you assess the risk and advise about appropriate fetal monitoring?

Is there evidence of pre-eclampsia (unlikely if not previously a problem, but check blood pressure and urine dipstick for protein)? Does the baby feel small (the perinatal mortality at term is 190/1000 for those < 5th centile, compared with 12/1000 for those > 10th centile)? And is there meconium-staining of the liquor? Labours using oxytocin or epidurals, or following a previous caesarean section, are also considered to be at higher risk. In the absence of these, it would be appropriate to use intermittent auscultation.

The blood pressure and urine are normal and the baby does not feel small. The liquor, however, is meconium stained. What is the significance of this?

Meconium staining of the liquor is associated with an increased chance of fetal distress. In addition, meconium is found below the baby's vocal cords postnatally in about one-third of cases in which it is present, and may give rise to the meconium aspiration syndrome. Clinical features of this syndrome range from mild neonatal tachypnoea to severe respiratory compromise. The incidence is probably unrelated to pH (and indeed the majority of babies with meconium aspiration syndrome are not acidotic at delivery) but the syndrome is more likely to be severe if there is associated acidosis. It is also more severe when the meconium is thick.

She is reluctant to agree to CTG, but accedes after considering your carefully worded advice. The CTG is shown in Fig. 53.1. What is your interpretation of this?

There is a baseline of 125 b.p.m. (normal range is 110–150 b.p.m.) with good beat-to-beat variability. Contractions are coming at approximately 1:3 min. There are accelerations and only one early deceleration which is unlikely to be of clinical significance.

Variability gives the best indication of fetal well-being, with normal being 10–25 b.p.m. The commonest reason for loss of baseline variability is the 'sleep' or 'quiet' phase of the fetal behavioural cycle, which may last up to 40 min. Loss of variability is also associated with prematurity, acidosis and drugs (e.g. opiates or benzodiazepines). The accelerations add extra reassurance. There should be at least two accelerations per 15 min with an amplitude greater than 15 b.p.m. lasting for at least 15 s, although there may be fewer accelerations in established labour.

A normal CTG in the presence of meconium provides reassurance, but an abnormal CTG becomes even more significant if meconium is present and should lower the threshold for investigation or intervention.

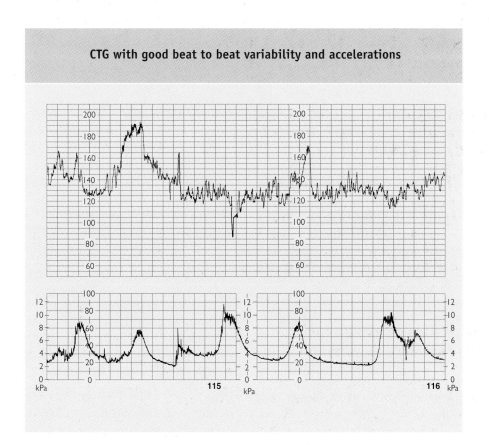

Fig. 53.1 *CTG with good beat-to-beat variability and accelerations. One early deceleration is seen.*

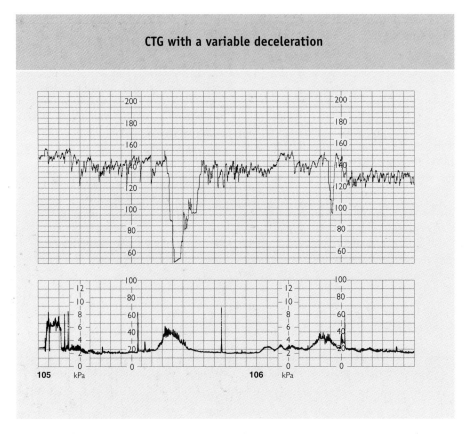

CTG with a variable deceleration

105   kPa

106   kPa

Fig. 53.2   *CTG with a variable deceleration.*

After 2 h, the cervix is 5 cm dilated; the CTG is shown in Fig 53.2. Describe the features of this trace and their significance.

The baseline is between 125 and 140 and, although there is still quite good beat-to-beat variability, there is a variable deceleration with no obvious shouldering. The contractions are more spread out, at 1:7 min.

Decelerations are defined as being of at least 15 b.p.m. and lasting for more than 15 s. 'Early' decelerations occur with contractions. If they occur more than 15 s after the contraction they are termed 'late'. 'Variable' contractions vary in both timing and shape:

- Early decelerations reflect increased vagal tone (intracranial pressure rises during a contraction) and are physiological.
- Variable decelerations may represent cord compression (e.g. in oligohydramnios) or acidosis. A small acceleration at the beginning and end of a deceleration (shouldering) suggests that the fetus is undistressed by the intermittent cord compression.
- Late decelerations suggest acidosis. Shallow late decelerations may be particularly ominous.

While this CTG might be acceptable in the presence of clear liquor, it is felt that further assessment is required. Feeling that control of this labour is slipping, she agrees to fetal blood sampling with some resignation. What is the value of fetal scalp pH measurement and how is it carried out?

Fetal blood sampling is used to establish further information following a suspicious CTG. Acidosis implies fetal hypoxaemia. A pH > 7.25 is normal, one between 7.20 and 7.25 is borderline, and one < 7.20 is abnormal.

The mother is placed in the lithotomy position with 15° lateral tilt (or left lateral position if approaching full dilatation). An amnioscope is inserted and the scalp dried with a sponge or swab. The scalp is then sprayed with ethyl chloride to induce hyperaemia and covered with a thin layer of paraffin jelly (so that the blood will form a blob and not run). Using a blade, a small nick is made in the scalp and the blob touched with a capillary tube so that it fills. If possible, three samples should be taken to ensure consistency of results.

The result is a pH of 7.27. An hour later, the cervix is 7 cm dilated; the CTG is as illustrated in Fig. 55.3. What features are shown?

There is a baseline of between 160 and 180 b.p.m. with absent beat-to-beat variability and persistent late decelerations. This, particularly in the presence of the meconium staining, is a highly suspicious CTG.

The scalp pH is repeated and this time is 7.15. What do you do?

The baby is showing significant evidence of distress and delivery would be considered appropriate. This is a major decision in a para 3 at 7 cm, as a caesarean section will be required, but the patient decides 'to put her baby first' and agrees. She is delivered of a baby boy weighing 3.2 kg with Apgar scores of 3 at 1 min, 5 at 5 min and 8 at 10 min.

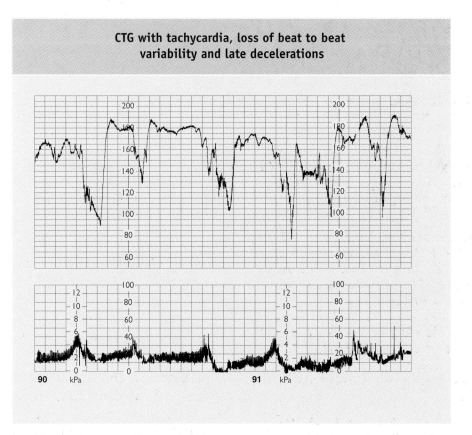

CTG with tachycardia, loss of beat to beat variability and late decelerations

Fig. 53.3 *CTG with tachycardia, loss of beat-to-beat variability and late decelerations.*

Table 53.1 *Neonatal encephalopathy grading*

Grade	Clinical features	Outcome
1	Hyperalert, decreased tone, jittery, dilated pupils	Usually resolve in 24 h
2	Lethargic, weak suck, fits	15–27% chance of severe sequelae
3	Flaccid, no suck, no Moro reflex, prolonged fits	Nearly 100% chance of severe sequelae

What are the implications of these scores on the baby's long-term outcome?

Apgar scores simply reflect the immediate level of resuscitation required and correlate poorly with long-term outcome. Of those with an Apgar score < 3 at 10 min, two-thirds die within 1 year. Of the survivors, 80% are normal.

Neonatal encephalopathy grading is a better guide to long-term outlook than Apgar scores (Table 53.1). The prognosis is generally good if the baby does not develop grade 3 neonatal encephalopathy, or if grade 2 neonatal encephalopathy lasts < 5 days. Further clinical evaluation may be available from EEG (incidence of death or handicap is low if normal or near normal), computed tomography (good prognosis if normal or only patchy hypodensities) or ultrasound (incidence of impairment correlates with intracerebral hypoechogenic areas of necrosis). The incidence of cerebral palsy in term infants has not changed with 'improved' obstetric care, and probably < 10% of cases are due to intrapartum events.

In this case there was no neonatal encephalopathy and the baby had a normal outcome.

Caesarean section

A 16 year old primigravida is admitted to the labour ward with regular uterine activity and a fully effaced, 5 cm dilated cervix. The CTG shows a normal heart rate but markedly reduced baseline variability with late decelerations. Thick fresh meconium is noted and the pH is 7.1 on fetal blood sampling.

A caesarean section is performed for fetal distress. How is this carried out?

Preparation includes intravenous access, group and save for possible transfusion, sodium citrate ± ranitidine (to reduce the incidence of Mendelson syndrome), appropriate thromboprophylaxis (Fig. 54.1) and antibiotic prophylaxis, anaesthesia (spinal, epidural or general) and catheterization. The table should be tilted 15° to the left side (to reduce aortocaval compression).

The uterine incision may be transverse (on the lower segment of the uterus) or vertical (classical). Lower uterine segment caesarean section is by far the most commonly used and has a lower rate of subsequent uterine rupture, together with better healing and fewer postoperative complications. A classical caesarean section will provide better access for a transverse lie following ruptured membranes, or with very vascular anterior placenta praevias, very preterm fetuses (particularly after spontaneous rupture of membranes), or large lower-segment fibroids. The chance of scar rupture in subsequent pregnancies following a vertical uterine incision is, however, much greater.

In this instance, a lower abdominal transverse incision is made, cutting through the fat and the rectus sheath to open the peritoneum. The bladder is freed and pushed down, and a transverse lower segment uterine incision made. The baby's head is encouraged through the incision with firm fundal pressure from the assistant (Wrigley forceps are occasionally required). If the baby is breech presentation, traction is applied to the pelvis by placing a finger behind each flexed hip, or if transverse, a foot should be identified and brought out to deliver the breech first (i.e. internal podalic version). After delivery, oxytocin is given i.v. stat and the placenta delivered after uterine contraction. Haemostasis is obtained with straight artery forceps, a check made to ensure that the uterus is empty and that there are no ovarian cysts, and the incision closed with two layers of dissolving suture to the uterus (e.g. Vicryl), one layer to the sheath and one layer to the skin.

Thromboprophylaxis for caesarean section

Low risk – Early mobilization and hydration

- Elective caesarean section – uncomplicated pregnancy and no other risk factors

Moderate risk – heparin (e.g. heparin 7500 iu b.i.d. or enoxaparin 20 mg daily) and compression stockings

- Age > 35 years
- Obesity (> 80 kg)
- Para 4 or more
- Gross varicose veins
- Current infection
- Pre-eclampsia
- Immobility prior to surgery (> 4 days)
- Major current illness, e.g. heart or lung disease; cancer; inflammatory bowel disease; nephrotic syndrome
- Emergency caesarean section in labour

High risk – heparin (e.g. heparin 7500 iu b.i.d. or 5000 iu t.i.d. or enoxaparin 40 mg daily) and compression stockings

- A patient with three or more moderate risk factors from above
- Extended major pelvic or abdominal surgery, e.g. caesarean hysterectomy
- Patients with a personal or family history of deep vein thrombosis; pulmonary embolism or thrombophilia; paralysis of lower limbs
- Patients with antiphospholipid antibody (cardiolipin antibody or lupus anticoagulant)

Fig. 54.1   *Thromboprophylaxis for caesarean section.*

Three years later, she is pregnant once more. Worried that she may require an intrapartum caesarean section again, she asks about the possibility of an elective caesarean. What are the pros and cons of this?

Caesarean section, particularly when carried out as an emergency in labour, carries a greater risk of morbidity and mortality than vaginal delivery, mostly from thromboembolic disease, haemorrhage and infection. Complications are minimized with the use of thromboprophylaxis, prophylactic antibiotics and regional anaesthesia. In subsequent pregnancies there is a small chance of intrapartum scar rupture. We must therefore ask 'What is the chance of a vaginal delivery this time around?'

In this instance, the caesarean section was for a non-recurrent cause, namely fetal distress. It would therefore be reasonable to plan for vaginal delivery this time, but the final decision should be a joint one between the patient and the obstetrician.

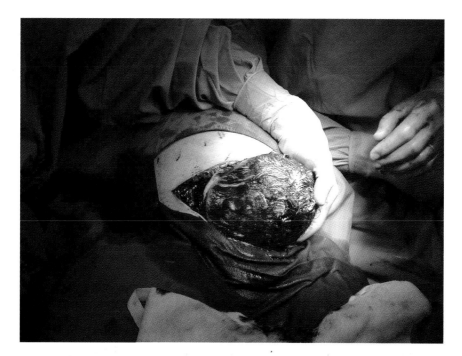

Fig. 54.2   *Caesarean section.*

Retained placenta

A 41 year old para 5 has a rapid labour at home and delivers a male infant in the bathroom; he begins to cry spontaneously. As a member of an obstetric 'flying squad', you arrive at the house following a emergency telephone call from her 14 year old daughter, who relays from her mother that the 'afterbirth is still inside'.

You arrive 25 min after the baby is born. What would your initial assessment involve?

One of the main worries is that the mother could be haemorrhaging. She is a grand multipara and may have an atonic uterus, although clearly the uterus must have been contracting effectively to deliver the baby half an hour previously. Look at the mother, the sheets, and the floor and ask about bleeding. Meantime ask the midwife to check that the baby is well. Check the mother's pulse and blood pressure and feel the uterine fundus (firm or flaccid?). Inspect the perineum. Is the placenta just siting at the introitus or, on gentle sterile vaginal examination, is it completely within the uterine cavity?

Her vital signs are normal and there has been minimal bleeding. You notice a lower abdominal transverse incision; on questioning the mother, you are told that this was for a caesarean section in her previous pregnancy, on account of a transverse lie. The midwife gives Syntometrine® as a prophylaxis against postpartum haemorrhage. What is Syntometrine?

This is a combination of 5 units Syntocinon (synthetic oxytocin) and 500 µg ergometrine (a natural amino acid alkaloid which acts as an alpha adrenoceptor antagonist) made up to a 1 ml solution. It causes the uterus to contact and should only be given after the baby has been born.

As she is in pain and as the uterus seems well contracted (making the risk of postpartum haemorrhage relatively small), you decide to attempt gentle delivery of the placenta. How should this be done?

Delivery of the placenta should never be forced before placental separation has occurred, in case the uterus is turned inside out (uterine inversion). Inversion is usually an iatrogenic third-stage complication occurring because of excessive traction on the cord, but can occur spontaneously with uterine atony or a congenitally abnormal uterus. Gentle traction should be applied to the cord while the other hand supports the uterus, holding it in a cephalic direction (Fig. 55.1). As the placenta passes through the introitus, pressure on the uterus is released. Care is then taken to ensure that the membranes are delivered completely and without tearing. The placenta should be examined to ensure that there are no missing pieces still in the uterine cavity.

The placenta does not come. What do you do next?

There is no definite length of time in which the placenta should be delivered, or after which it is termed 'a retained placenta'. You should transfer your patient to hospital in case a manual removal under general anaesthetic or regional block becomes necessary.

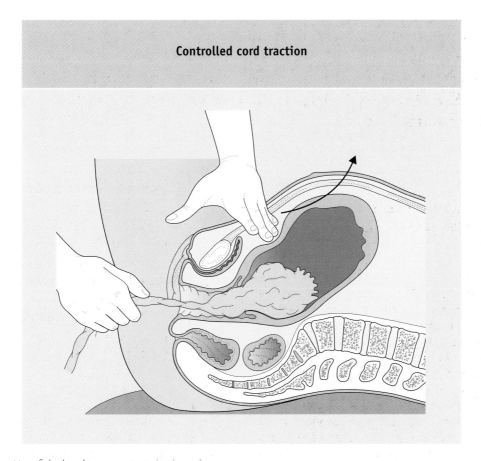

Controlled cord traction

Fig. 55.1 *Use of the hand to prevent uterine inversion.*

She arrives on the labour ward 60 min after the baby has been born. What next?

Send blood for cross-match and establish intravenous access. It is worth another gentle attempt at continuous cord traction. This, however, is unsuccessful.

There is evidence that delaying theatre for up to an hour after delivery (in the absence of bleeding) will increase the chance of delivering the placenta without intervention. In this case the baby has been out for 75 min and you therefore decide to transfer to theatre for a 'manual removal of placenta'.

How is this done and what are the potential problems?

After blood has been cross-matched and is available on the labour ward, arrange either a general anaesthetic or regional block (e.g. spinal anaesthetic). The patient is placed in the lithotomy position and, with asepsis, a last attempt is made with gentle cord traction and uterine support. If this fails, a hand is inserted through the cervical os (the os may need to be redilated with the fingers) and the fingers then used to separate the placenta from the uterine wall (Fig. 55.2). Care must be taken to avoid uterine perforation, particularly at the site of

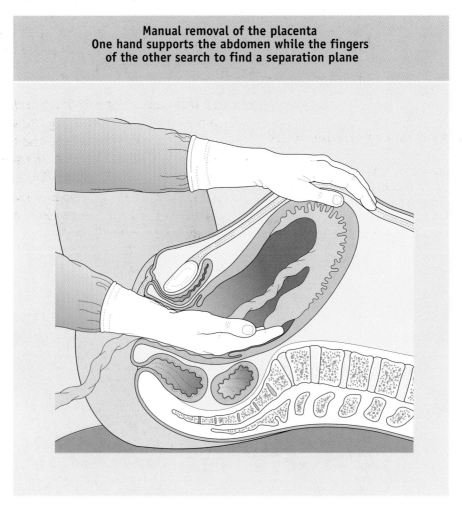

Manual removal of the placenta
One hand supports the abdomen while the fingers
of the other search to find a separation plane

Fig. 55.2 *Manual removal of the placenta.*

a previous caesarean section scar, as in this case. There are also risks of postpartum haemorrhage (give further oxytocin or Syntometrine after the placenta is delivered), infection (give antibiotics) and uterine inversion.

Rarely the placenta may be 'morbidly adherent', termed placenta accreta. This may be due to placenta increta (penetration of the placenta into the myometrium) or placenta percreta (penetration through the myometrium to serosa or beyond) and is more likely to occur if the placenta overlies a previous caesarean scar. The adherent placenta cannot be separated digitally and further management depends on the amount of bleeding. If minimal, the placenta should be left in situ and the patient warned of the high probability of secondary postpartum haemorrhage, which often occurs 10–14 days later. If there is bleeding, further oxytocics may be tried, but if she has completed her family, hysterectomy is the treatment of choice. If not, additional oxytocics and internal iliac artery ligation are options.

How would you manage uterine inversion?

If complete uterine inversion occurs, there is often severe lower abdominal pain and profound hypotension (neurogenic in origin). It may be possible to replace the uterus immediately, followed by an intravenous oxytocic to encourage contraction. If this is not possible, start antishock measures with intravenous access and colloid. Then:

- If the placenta is still attached and easily removable, remove it once the shock is corrected, ideally under general anaesthetic.
- If unsuccessful, use hydrostatic reduction (O'Sullivan method). Exclude perforation by clinical inspection. The inverted uterus is held within the vagina by the operator and the introitus sealed with the two hands of an assistant. Infuse 2 litres of warm saline rapidly (e.g. with 1000 ml bags of saline through a urological Y giving set, or through a funnel and tube as for a stomach washout, or using anaesthetic gas tubing).
- Once corrected, give Syntometrine 1 ml i.m. stat.
- If all this fails, consider a vaginal or abdominal surgical approach, with division of the cervix.

In this case, although the placenta is anterior and just overlying the previous scar, manual removal under general anaesthetic is uneventful. The scar is confirmed to be intact by digital examination, there is no postpartum haemorrhage and the mother returns home the following day.

Postpartum haemorrhage

You are the most senior obstetrician working in a small rural hospital with good laboratory facilities. It is the middle of winter and the hospital has been snowbound by a blizzard. The snow has also brought down the telephone cables, effectively cutting off all communication. A 21 year old primigravida has just had a spontaneous vertex delivery following a 14 h labour, and you are called because of a 'brisk' postpartum haemorrhage.

What are the causes of postpartum haemorrhage?

There are three main causes:

- Uterine atony (the majority).
- Genital tract trauma, which may occur sponta- neously or following instrumental delivery (less common).
- Coagulation disorders (rare).

How would you manage the situation?

Assess the amount of bleeding by 'eyeballing' the bed and the floor. This is notoriously inaccu- rate, but gathering up the mess into a measuring container is impractical in the acute situation. Check that Syntometrine has been given. Look to see if the mother is pale and ask for pulse and blood pressure to be checked. Feel the uterus. Is it firm (i.e. well contracted) or flaccid (atonic)?

The uterus is atonic. What would you do?

Ask a midwife to 'rub a contraction up' firmly and carry on yourself to make a brief assessment of the perineum for obvious trauma. Establish intra- venous access with initially one (and as soon as possible two) large-bore cannulas. Give more oxy- tocin (e.g. 10 units i.v. stat). Send blood for haemoglobin, haematocrit, platelets and clotting and cross-match 6 units of red cell concentrate. Run colloid in fast (e.g. Haemaccel®, Gelofusine® or stable plasma solution — but not dextran because of the risk of anaphylaxis).

The placenta is retained (see also p. 168) but fortunately is easily removed with

gentle continuous cord traction. The bleeding continues and the uterus still feels atonic. What would you do next?

Call the anaesthetist. Ensure that uterine massage is continuing. Give further oxytocics to encourage uterine contraction. This may be in the form of oxytocin 20 units i.v. stat, ergometrine 0.5 mg i.v. stat or carboprost (Hemabate®) 250 mg i.m. (*not i.v.*). Set up an intravenous infusion of sytocinon.

Forty minutes have elapsed since delivery and you estimate the bleeding at 1500-2000 ml. The pulse is 120 b.p.m., the blood pressure 80/40 mmHg and the patient looks pale and drowsy. The initial clotting screen is normal and the haemoglobin 9.6 g/dl. She has had 1000 ml of colloid and the first unit of red cell concentrate is running. The uterus now feels more firm, but bleeding continues.

Continue with intravenous fluids, both colloid and red cell concentrate, to maintain the intravascular volume. Insert a urethral catheter, with an hourly urimeter to assess renal function. The fact that the uterus is firm and bleeding is continuing raises the possibility of genital tract trauma. To examine this properly, particularly the cervix, a general anaesthetic is required.

Under anaesthesia and with asepsis, examine the introitus and vagina for lacerations. Explore the uterine cavity digitally, looking for retained pieces of placenta, or (rarely) for signs of rupture. Identify the cervix, grasp it with atraumatic forceps and carefully check all the way around for tears. If any vaginal or cervical tear is identified, it should be sutured.

The uterus is empty and a small vaginal tear is repaired. She has received 2500 ml clear fluid as both crystalloid and colloid, and 5 units of red cell concentrate. The

pulse is still 120 b.p.m. with a blood pressure of 80/40 mmHg. Two hours have now elapsed and the uterus remains well contracted. The bleeding, which seems to be coming from within the uterus itself, continues. What would you do next?

Send off a further clotting screen and insert a CVP line to guide fluid replacement. Also check urea, electrolytes (large blood transfusions may lead to hyperkalaemia following red cell lysis) and calcium (the sodium citrate preservative binds calcium, leading to hypocalcaemia). The results of the full blood count and clotting screen are as follows:

	Result	Normal values
Hb (g/dl)	6.4	10-13
Platelets ($\times 10^9$/l)	35	150-400
APTT (s)	74	Control 31
INR (s)	54	Control 12
Fibrinogen (g/dl)	<0.5	2-6
Fibrin degradation products (mg/l)	8-16	<0.25

What does this signify and what needs to be done?

The patient has DIC. In this condition there is rapid conversion of fibrinogen to fibrin (a large polypeptide), due to stimulation of the intrinsic and extrinsic clotting pathways (hence the raised APTT, INR and low fibrinogen). At the same time there is rapid breakdown of fibrin (by the enzyme plasmin) to smaller amino acid chains (hence the increased fibrin degradation products). The end-result is a reduction in available clotting factors and an increased bleeding tendency.

The clotting factors need to be replaced. This may be in the form of fresh frozen plasma or cryoprecipitate (which is prepared from fresh frozen plasma and is a rich source of fibrinogen, factor VIII and von Willebrand factor). While low platelets in the asymptomatic patient do not require treatment, this patient is bleeding and it would be reasonable to give platelet concentrate as well.

Despite correcting the coagulopathy, the bleeding continues. The pulse is 140 b.p.m. and the blood pressure barely maintained at 70/30 mmHg. What would you do next?

Despite all these conservative measures, the bleeding is continuing and is threatening the patient's life. Surgery is now indicated. Internal iliac artery ligation may be of some use, but hysterectomy (or subtotal hysterectomy) is the treatment of choice. This is, of course, a radical step in this young primigravida and should only be carried out when all other options have been exhausted. The other option is for radiological internal iliac artery embolization (Fig. 56.1), but this is unlikely to be available in a small rural hospital.

A subtotal hysterectomy is carried out and the patient recovers. Could this postpartum haemorrhage have been predicted or prevented?

This patient was at relatively low risk of postpartum haemorrhage, although her labour had

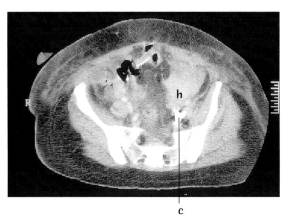

Fig. 56.1 *The left internal iliac artery has been embolized, and the embolization coils **c** are seen as the bright area to the right of the image (patient's left). There is a large pelvic haematoma **h** above this.*

been prolonged. It is more common in grand multiparity, multiple pregnancy, fibroids, placenta praevia, following an antepartum haemorrhage and in those with a past history of postpartum haemorrhage. None of these applied.

Prophylactic oxytocics (see Syntometrine, p. 168) do reduce the risk of postpartum haemorrhage, and these had been given. The staff were also quick to recognize the problem and summon help, so that, on balance, it is unlikely that this could have been prevented. It may be worth excluding a congenital coagulation defect at a later stage (e.g. von Willebrand disease).

Further reading

Boylan P 2002 Active Management of Labour, 4th edn. Mosby, London

Chamberlain G, Steer P 2001 Turnbull's Obstetrics, 3rd edn. Churchill Livingstone, Edinburgh

de Swiet M 2002 Medical Disorders in Obstetric Practice. Blackwell Science, London

Greer I, Cameron I, Kitchener H, Prentice A 2000 Mosby's Color Atlas and Text of Obstetrics and Gynaecology. Mosby, London

Magowan B 2000 Churchill's Pocketbook of Obstetrics and Gynaecology, 2nd edn. Churchill Livingstone, Edinburgh

Shaw R W, Souter P W, Stanton S L 1997 Gynaecology, 2nd edn. Churchill Livingstone, Edinburgh

Smith N C, Smith A P M 2001 Obstetric Ultrasound Made Easy. Churchill Livingstone, Edinburgh

Thomson A J 2000 Antenatal Disorder for the MRCOG and Beyond. RCOG Press, London

Index